CLEANSING
made simple

♦♦♦

Cheryl Townsley

LFH Publishing
P.O. Box 3871, Littleton, CO 80161

Graphics: Nick Zellinger
Text Design: Theresa Frank

This publication is designed to provide accurate and
authoritative information in regard to the subject matter
covered. It is sold with the understanding that the author
and the publisher are not engaged in rendering legal,
medical, or other professional service. If medical services or other expert consultation is required, the services
of a competent professional should be sought.

Townsley, Cheryl
        Cleansing made simple /
    Cheryl Townsley
        Includes bibliographical references
        ISBN 0-9644566-6-4
        1. Toxicology. 2. Health. 3. Nutrition. I. Title.

For information contact:

LFH Publishing
8122 Southpark Lane, Suite 114
Littleton, CO 80120
For ordering information, refer to the last page.

Printed in the United States of America

CONTENTS
✦✦✦

CONTENTS
✦✦✦

What once was so dirty, hopeless and defiled ...
is now becoming clean and whole.
Clean or unclean,
the choice is yours.

As the end of the age draws nigh,
begin to cleanse
from the inside out.

Be the whole person
God created YOU to be!

ACKNOWLEDGMENTS
✦✦✦

Just when I think there are no more words to write, another book bubbles forth from the inside of me. Each time, our team demonstrates excellence in presenting our audience with a book that will help them obtain health — in a practical and affordable manner.

Thanks to Theresa Frank for being one of the most intelligent, creative people I have the privilege to know. Her attention to detail in formatting this book has produced a real winner.

Thanks to Debbie Blissard and Lory Floyd for proofing the text and helping make my ideas understandable to our readers. Their attention to each "i" and "t" makes this as close to error-free as humanly possible.

Thanks to Nick Zellinger for his creativity on the cover. Nick combines art with computer skills to produce excellence on the packaging of the printed page.

Thanks to Forest and Anna for supporting me during another creative splurge. Molding ideas into functional concepts takes time and energy. They provide the support, encouragement and love to allow my creativity to flow unhindered.

Last, but not least, thanks to the ever-growing LFH team that provides skills, expertise and gifts that far surpass the work of one person. I may write the words, but God has provided a team and the "life" that brings a book to fruition.

INTRODUCTION
✦✦✦

Being a Type A, choleric, driver, firstborn, German perfectionist, I certainly had no time to be sick. I had a job (or two or three) to do. For more than three decades my ability to perform served me quite well, or so I thought. I excelled at business, made large amounts of money and appeared to be successful.

By my mid-thirties, change set in. After a difficult pregnancy, I found my health to be challenged in more ways than I could count. Decades of stress, poor nutrition, lack of exercise, and the constant pressure to perform and excel had robbed me of my health reserves and left me bankrupt. That accumulated toll had occurred behind the scenes. Pregnancy merely raised the curtain on a performance I had no desire to witness. The ticket to that performance was vastly expensive — it almost cost me my life.

At the ripe age of 35, I became overweight, sick, severely depressed and suicidal. Nine months after my last suicide attempt, I was introduced to a nutritionist. Hope was being birthed in me.

Through his expertise and my curiosity, I began one of the most fascinating times of discovery and growth that I have ever experienced. The bottom line of his advice can be summarized in the phrase, "Cleanse and build!"

It was time for me to cleanse my body of accumulated toxins and build my health and reserves. At the time I had no understanding or comprehension of his words. Cleanse? Did that mean I was dirty? Had I not been so sick, I just might have been offended by that comment!

Build? How could a person build health? If you're sick, you obviously just need the right pill to make the problem disappear. Alas, as with millions of my American counterparts, I had much to learn and most of what I thought I knew was incorrect. I knew so little about how to steward this precious creation called Cheryl Townsley.

This education process has made me a student of choices and consequences. I have learned that there are consequences to my choices in every area of life, including health. After years of simply choosing what was convenient and easy with no thought to my health, I learned that convenience had its price. It was now time to actually learn how to care for my body and correct the damage that had been done in the name of convenience. I had to open the operations manual and begin to apply some effort to restore and build my health.

As my knowledge level has increased, so has my wisdom. In the arena of health, I have not stopped with mere knowledge, since it has no value unless it is applied. It is in the actual application of health principles that we can produce the good fruit of health.

It is from the experience of seeing my health restored that I share with you what I have learned. I have no desire to simply add to your knowledge. I desire most of all to see you learn wisdom. For years I hungered for knowledge, but found only mental constipation. Now, I am beginning to understand that wisdom is far more valuable.

Unlike knowledge, wisdom is:

- ◆ the ability to know when and how to apply information, and
- ◆ knowing what question to ask and of whom to ask it.

To restore my health I had to learn how to apply what I knew and to ask what I did not know — of the right people. To determine who those "right" people are, I have had to identify and evaluate the fruit of "health" in their lives. Are they healthy? Do they live what they preach? What do I look for? I look for a life-style of health.

Our nutritionist began the process. He taught us the importance of cleansing — getting out toxins and that which retards health. He also taught us how to build — bring in the new that's needed to build a health body. I continue to appreciate the value of a "cleansing and building" approach to health. This process effects my entire life — physical, mental, emotional, spiritual, financial and relational. Health is not a destination, it is a process that will last your entire life.

As you walk through the pages of *Cleansing made simple*, I pray that you will take the information and strategies, digest them, convert them into wisdom *and* apply them. It is in the application that you will begin to experience the fruit of health.

The very word *health*, if traced to its Hebrew roots, comes from the word *shalom*. Shalom is peace, or to have safety in your mind, body and estate. What you are today and what you pass on to future generations lays the foundation for peace. This kind of peace supersedes the stress of our modern age.

Enter into the shalom of health. Learn how to cleanse your body and your life of the toxins that rob you of peace and health. But, most importantly, learn to apply and refine what you learn from those who have a lifestyle rich in peace and health.

As you cleanse out the impurities in your life — body, soul and spirit — and become refined, you will become a vessel of purest gold. I bless you to be the whole person God created you to be! As the prophet Jeremiah said,

> "For I (God) know the thoughts and plans that I have for you, thoughts and plans for welfare and *peace* (health) and not for evil, to give you *hope* in your final outcome."

ONE
A HEALTHY BODY
✦✦✦

Modern technology has extended our life spans, but often at the cost of chronic disease. These diseases can manifest as autoimmune diseases (i.e., heart disease, diabetes, multiple sclerosis, fibromyalgia, arthritis, etc.), depression or cancer. Current statistics are alarming and ever increasing. As the baby boomers reach retirement age in the next 15 to 30 years, these chronic diseases will only escalate. If you are doing nothing to prevent these diseases, then it is only a matter of time before you are one of these alarming statistics.

WELLNESS DEFINED

In order to know where we are headed, we need to have a working definition of health. Since a picture is worth a thousand words, let's paint a picture of health for our definition. From this vision, you can begin to compare your current health status with what is possible.

Many people have the image that health is "being free of cancer and being skinny." With their acceptance of this incomplete definition, many people miss out on the more practical, big-picture of true health. While sitting in the office of a health care provider, I read an excellent definition of wellness. Let me share this definition with you.

Good health means much more than being free of disease. Here are 13 symptoms of good health:

- Having energy for all required activities and a surplus for recreation.
- Having good appetite and digestion.
- Having daily, comfortable elimination.
- Having healthy eyes, shiny hair and radiant skin.
- Having a flexible body and stable emotions.
- Maintaining good memory and clear thinking.
- Being free from anxiety, worry and depression.
- Being able to enjoy activities, recreation and even overall relaxation.
- Having good communication skills to express your innermost thoughts and feelings.
- Participating in regular, spontaneous outbreaks of humor and laughter.
- Having healthy esteem of self and others.
- Having a personal relationship with the Living God.
- Being free from dis-ease.

This is a far cry from the perception that health is being skinny and free of cancer. Health is a daily walk — a lifestyle based on wise choices, moment by moment, for the rest of your life. The freedom from sickness and dis-ease brings even more exciting "side effects."

IMPORTANT BODY PARTS

We have all heard the advertising adage, "parts is parts." However, not all parts are the same. Your body is comprised of many systems, organs, glands and metabolic functions. In order to understand health and the role of cleansing, we must more fully understand how the body works. The body is a miraculous creation that is fearfully and awesomely made. Join me as we tour the body from top to bottom.

SKIN

The skin is our largest cleansing organ. It can eliminate more cellular waste than the colon and kidneys combined. The skin is comprised of an outer layer (the epidermis) and an inner layer (the dermis).

The outer layer of the skin is replenished every 14 days. The health of the epidermis determines how easily chemicals can penetrate the skin. Skin color is determined by melanin, which protects against ultraviolet and visible light and helps quench free radicals. Epidermal cells produce lipids (fats such as cholesterol and essential fatty acids), which help waterproof the body and help it hold together.

The dermis consists of collagen and elastin, which give skin its elasticity and strength. The sweat glands and hair follicles are also contained in the dermis. Sweat glands not only "sweat," they also help us regulate our internal temperature.

If the skin is not adequately lubricated by essential fatty acids, then solvents and other chemicals can easily penetrate the skin. Skin absorbs harmful elements based on the following conditions:

- ♦ Oily solutions penetrate the skin more easily.
- ♦ Elements that are slightly water- and fat-soluble penetrate the skin more easily.
- ♦ Wet skin allows for water-soluble elements to enter the skin more easily.
- ♦ Hotter temperatures allow for elements to enter the skin more easily.
- ♦ Elements can enter the body via hair follicles.
- ♦ Injured skin allows for easier penetration.

RESPIRATORY TRACT

Our respiratory tract includes the nose, pharynx, larynx, trachea and lungs. Air enters through the nose and travels across the trachea. The trachea branches into the right and left lungs. Our lungs receive oxygen, which is sent to the cells via the capillaries. They also expel the metabolic waste — carbon dioxide.

Some similar forms of respiratory tract diseases are asthma, bronchitis and emphysema. Asthma manifests as wheezing or breathing difficulty. Bronchitis shows up as inflammation of the bronchial tubes. Emphysema impairs lung elasticity. The lungs are most impacted by our environment.

The lungs use mucous and cilia to help protect against harmful inhalants. When the system can trap these elements, it removes them through sneezing and coughing. Mucous is a secretion that forms a lining throughout the respiratory tract. Cilia are hair-like projections that beat 1,000 times per minute and help remove foreign elements from the lungs. Cilia are dependent on the right balance of mucous.

LYMPH

Lymph is part of the lymphatic system, which serves as a transport system. It transports nutrients to the cells and exports toxins. As an exporter, it works like a drainage system, eliminating matter that has escaped the bloodstream or was too large to enter the blood. Once the offending matter is caught by the lymph nodes, it is attacked by the immune system.

Unlike the blood, which is pumped, lymph must be stimulated. Excellent methods of stimulation include skin brushing, massage and jumping on rebounders (miniature trampolines). Water consumption is critical for lymph formation and flow.

GI TRACT

The gastrointestinal (GI) tract includes the mouth, esophagus, stomach, small intestine, large intestine and rectum. Other glandular organs, such as the salivary glands, liver, gallbladder and pancreas impact the GI tract. The purpose of the GI tract is to digest food and get it into a form that the body can use and assimilate. The digestive organs manufacture nearly one gallon of juice per day to help with digestion and assimilation. Emotions greatly impact the ability of the GI tract to digest food.

The GI tube runs from the mouth to the anus, or about five yards. When food is eaten, it mixes with saliva (containing amylase, a carbohydrate digesting enzyme), which begins the digestive process. The esophagus serves as a tube to move the food from the mouth to the stomach via swallowing.

The stomach mixes the food with hydrochloric acid, mucous and digestive juices. Pepsin helps digest proteins and gastrin helps release the appropriate amounts of hydrochloric acid. The result of these juices on food produces "chyme." With adequate amounts of hydrochloric acid, any ingested bacteria is killed.

From the stomach, "chyme" (or partially digested food) travels to the small intestine. Enzymes from the pancreas begin to digest the "chyme" into fatty acids, simple sugars and amino acids. These substances cross the intestinal wall and enter the blood and lymph.

The remainder of our food enters the large intestine, and is primarily water, minerals and undigested matter. The large intestine removes water and removes the waste through bowel movements called feces.

The colon is part of the large intestine. Proper levels of friendly bacteria are critical for a healthy colon. Having adequate amounts of good bacteria, "good critters," helps decrease the growth of "bad critters" (i.e., yeast, fungus, parasites and bacteria). The total weight of these "good critters" should be approximately three to five pounds.

Poor assimilation throughout the GI tract (i.e., leaky gut) can produce deficiencies, allergies and immune problems. An overgrowth of yeast in the GI tract can lead to candida. The following disorders may occur with leaky gut:

- ♦ irritable bowel syndrome
- ♦ Crohn's disease
- ♦ rheumatoid arthritis

LIVER

The liver is a dome-shaped gland that sits at the lower edge of your right rib cage. It weights about five pounds and is the largest gland in the body. It uses over 12 percent of our total energy supply. Over 1½ quarts of blood flows through the liver each minute.

The body can function without the colon or stomach, but not the liver. It is the body's primary filter and detoxification site for the blood. If the bowel does not contain and eliminate harmful elements, then they are reabsorbed into the blood. The toxins are then sent back to the liver. This puts a large burden on the liver.

The liver has several functions, including:

♦ Carbohydrate, vitamin and mineral storage.
♦ Fat, protein and carbohydrate metabolization.
♦ Hormone and foreign chemical metabolization.
♦ Synthesizing blood proteins.
♦ Assimilation and storage of fat-soluble vitamins.
♦ Bile formation.

KIDNEYS
These paired organs are primary excretory organs and lie on the abdominal wall, one on each side of the backbone. They are shaped like beans. They filter the blood and drain wastes, mostly from protein digestion. They help to maintain the body's pH, calcium and electrolyte balances. They also help eliminate foreign matter from the body.

The kidneys receive 25 percent of the body's total blood volume, causing high exposure to chemicals in the blood. Of the blood filtered, 0.1 percent becomes urine. Approximately 10 percent of the normal resting oxygen is used by the kidneys.

Urine is carried from the kidneys via the ureter to the bladder. Its walls are smooth muscles that unfold to hold increasing urine amounts. When the bladder is full, it contracts. Urine then flows, as a voluntary action, through the urethra out of the body.

BALANCING THE BODY
The key to health is the ability of the body to stay in homeostasis or balance. The two extremes that cause the most imbalance are deficiency and congestion. A deficiency occurs when we are not obtaining enough nutrients to meet our bodily needs. Congestion,

an excessive intake of too much food, stimulants (caffeine, alcohol, nicotine, refined sugar) and/or chemicals, can lead to impaired elimination and/or exhaustion stemming from the congestion of too much food intake.

The body needs to be balanced in many areas.

AREAS NEEDING BALANCE

BIOCHEMICAL

Life in the body exists due to hundreds of biochemical reactions every second. Every activity in the body, from neurotransmitter communication in the brain and nervous system to hormonal messages require biochemical reactions. The body must also be in pH balance (acid to alkaline) for detox pathways to stay open. Disease lives in an acid environment; it will not live in an alkaline environment. This is why the pH of the body is so crucial. Detox pathways are the "highways and byways" the body uses to empty the trash — toxins — leftover from biochemical reactions and other metabolic activities.

ELECTRICAL

The body is an electrical system from the brain to the muscles. Intake of minerals effects this electrical system. Electron transfers occurs in every biochemical reaction of the body. Without a balance in the power source, (i.e., minerals), the electrical demands in the body can surpass the electrical supply. This leads to a power shortage, which can manifest as MS, fibromyalgia or other weak muscle disorders.

EMOTIONAL

Many people do not realize that unresolved emotions (i.e., anger, fear, unforgiveness, guilt) actually convert to a chemical reaction and are stored in various parts of the body. Two of the most offending emotions are fear and anger. Nurturing, love and peace are necessary to balance any negative emotions.

ENERGY

The breakdown of matter (in other words, food) in the body releases energy to enable the cells to do their job. When this system is out of balance, both the body's temperature and energy levels are effected. This entire area of energy is called the body's metabolism. Metabolism runs our thermostats (temperature) and controls our energy reserves.

ENVIRONMENTAL

Common environmental pollutants add stress to the body. We often overlook pollution, pesticides, electromagnetic fields, etc., and how they impact our bodies. When our environment is out of balance, our bodies are also out of balance.

ENZYMES

Enzymes are the spark plugs of the body. They are essential for biochemical reactions to occur such as digestion and assimilation. Without enzymes we do not digest our food, which results in indigestion, excess weight and allergies. Enzymes also help in the digestion and assimilation of nutritional supplements. A well-fueled car will still go nowhere without spark plugs. So it is with your body. Without enzymes, your energy is depleted and food is not well utilized.

HORMONES

Hormones carry communications throughout the body. They impact metabolism, circulation, reproduction, stress, electrolytes and water balance. Hormones are much more than estrogen, progesterone and testosterone. Hormones are vital to the body parts communicating with each other.

MAGNETIC

Our brains produce a steady magnetic field. Imbalances can impact our body clocks, sleep patterns and muscles.

MENTAL
Mental health requires a balance of work and relaxation. All work and no play makes for a stressed person, which opens the door to fatigue and disease.

NUTRITION
The body must have a balance of vitamins, minerals, amino acids, proteins, carbohydrates and fats to be fully nourished and fully functional.

PSYCHOLOGICAL
The body must balance emotions with a logical mind. Unrestrained emotions or demanding logic can break down our psychological balance and lead to psychological problems that can also manifest as physical health problems.

RELATIONAL
Balance in relationships effects our emotions and sense of overall well-being. Having the ability to freely receive and give allows us to be well rounded in our relationships with others. Being either an "abuser" or a "victim" creates imbalances that negatively impact a person's health.

SPIRITUAL
We are created as a spirit, soul (mind, will and emotions) and body being. All three entities must be in balance. God created us with a purpose and to have fellowship with Him. Having a purpose or destiny gives life meaning.

STRUCTURE
The skeleton gives the body its plumb line. When the spine (or back bone) is in alignment, the rest of the body's bones, organs and systems can be in structural alignment. Just as a level foundation keeps a wall in alignment, so the spine keeps the body in alignment.

The real miracle of the body is that regardless of how we treat it (or mistreat, as the case may be), it manages to function. In order to be healthy, each of these systems must be in good working order and be in balance.

Harmful elements can enter the body at any of these access points. The next stop on our body tour is the identification of these harmful elements ... toxins.

TWO
WHAT ARE TOXINS?
✦✦✦

We have briefly surveyed this amazing creation called the human body. As we enter into the next millennium, we carry with us more chronic dis-ease and sickness than ever before. The connection between toxicity and increased dis-ease is obvious. As the toxic load has increased on the body, so has the body's response to the pressure. That response is sickness, dis-ease, loss of energy and premature death.

TOXINS DEFINED
A toxin is a substance that creates irritation or causes other harmful effects in the body. Toxins undermine our health by stressing our bodily systems and their metabolic functions. Toxicity occurs when we are out of balance in any of the aforementioned areas or when the body no longer has the ability to maintain health on its own. Toxins are the building blocks of disease and premature death.

Toxins cause the body to be defiled. *Defiled* is an interesting word: it is composed of "de" and "file." A file is anything that is in order. When "de" is added to file, it means to take out of order or out of balance. In fact, the *Webster Dictionary* defines defile as to make filthy. An intake of toxins defiles the body; it makes the body filthy.

SOURCES OF TOXINS

Toxins usually enter a person through four different access points. They can be absorbed through the skin, inhaled through the respiratory tract, ingested through the mouth into the GI tract and/or submitted as unresolved thoughts or emotions.

Numerous toxins can enter through these ports. Let's briefly review the more common sources of toxins and/or bodily toxicity that can negatively impact the body.

Sources of Toxins

♦ unresolved emotions	♦ soil depletion
♦ green produce	♦ tainted meat
♦ tainted dairy	♦ polluted water
♦ polluted environment	♦ lack of enzymes
♦ lack of fiber	♦ refined sugar
♦ damaged fats	♦ caffeine
♦ inadequate chewing	♦ stress

As we examine each of these toxins, do not become overwhelmed. The goal is not to add depression to the list. Your ignorance does not change the negative impact of toxins on your body. However, with knowledge, you can be informed, equipped and encouraged to change the future of your health status.

UNRESOLVED EMOTIONS

Health editor Emrika Padus writes, "It is estimated that 90 percent of all physical problems have psychological roots .... A growing body of evidence indicates that virtually every ill that can befall the body is influenced, for better or worse, by our emotions."[1]

---

[1] Emrika Padus & ed. of *Prevention Magazine, The Complete Guide to Your Emotions and Health.* p. 563

The two most devastating emotions appear to be fear and anger. Research has shown that unresolved fear can manifest as asthma, respiratory problems and upper chest tightness. Anger can settle in the liver. Other unresolved emotions that have been linked to health problems include:

♦ bitterness → gall bladder
♦ guilt → shoulder problems
♦ control or hatred → colon
♦ loneliness → aches
♦ suppression → allergies
♦ hostility or unforgiveness → arthritis
♦ inadequate finances → lower back problems
♦ resentment → candida
♦ despair → chronic fatigue
♦ nervousness → coughs
♦ need for protection → weight
♦ stress → headaches
♦ grief → lupus
♦ inflexibility → multiple sclerosis
♦ irritation → skin problems
♦ insecurity → stomach problems

The list can go on and on. It is important to realize that these problems may not be impacted by these emotional issues. However, it is usually helpful to at least examine emotional roots when health problems manifest. To ignore emotional roots when cleansing minimizes the impact of emotions in our life.

SOIL DEPLETION
Over the last one hundred years, we have sought to maximize production of crops on less soil and in less time. As a result, our soil has become depleted of its naturally occurring minerals. Even the Department of Agriculture acknowledges that our soil has fewer minerals today than at the turn of the century.

Rutgers University did research that was published as the Firma Bear Report on the depletion of minerals from our soil. This report states that soil microbes decompose and make minerals available to our plants. Many commercial crops are grown on dead, depleted soil and are fed by synthetic chemicals, which makes the plants weak and less healthy.

Studies show that insects selectively attack weak, unhealthy plants and leave healthy ones alone. As a result, commercial growers rely on pesticides to protect the crops. Conversely, organic produce is grown on healthy soil without synthetic chemicals. It offers greater nutritional value and higher mineral and trace elements content.

This chart shows how much more of each of the nutrients the organically grown food has over the conventionally grown food (i.e., organic snap beans have 2.6 times more calcium than do their conventional counterparts).

	CALCIUM	MAGNESIUM	POTASSIUM	IRON
Snap Beans	2.6	4.0	3.4	22.7
Cabbage	3.4	2.8	2.8	4.7
Lettuce	4.4	3.8	3.3	57.3
Tomatoes	5.1	13.2	2.5	1938.0
Spinach	2.0	4.3	3. 1	83.3

Since most Americans are not eating organic produce, they are lacking many minerals and trace elements. The result is a negative impact on the brain, bones, muscles and other parts of the body.

GREEN PRODUCE

With the advent of shipping, we now have the ability to eat from anywhere in the world anytime we want it. However, with shipping comes a problem. In order for the produce to appear pleasing to our eyes in the store, it must be picked green and shipped before it ripens and becomes blemished.

It is the vine-ripening process that enhances taste and creates the phytochemicals. Phytochemicals are nutrients plants make as a by-product of the vine-ripening process. Consequently, most of the produce in commercial grocery stores has minimal taste and less nutrition than it could have if it had been ripened on the vine.

We know about the importance of plants in providing vitamins and minerals. Since the increase of cancer, the American Cancer Society has regularly informed us of the need for daily intake of fruits and vegetables. In fact, the Surgeon General (1988) linked nutritional problems to five of the 10 leading causes of death in the U. S. (heart disease, cancer, strokes, non-insulin diabetes and arteriosclerosis).

Research has further shown the need for phytochemicals or "plant" based nutrition. Phytochemicals have been defined as the chemicals found in plants that are not vitamins or minerals yet are essential for health. The USDA, in its food pyramid, recommends 3 – 5 servings of vegetables and 2 – 4 servings of fruits per day.

According to research, only about 20 percent of Americans eat this amount of fruits and vegetables.[2] That means 80 percent do not eat enough fruits and vegetables and are susceptible to disease. Not only is most of the produce we consume not organic, it is usually picked green and is missing valuable phytochemicals.

Phytochemicals only occur in vine-ripened produce. Phytochemicals are the nutrients designed to be in plants by our Creator. When we shortchange that vine-ripening process because of our hurry to get merchandise to market, we minimize the nutritional value of the produce. Produce becomes mere merchandise to be displayed instead of consumed. If it is not attractive enough, we wax it, gas it or otherwise "improve" it. Sad to say, this merchandising effort destroys the most valuable aspect of produce — phytochemicals that produce life and health.

TAINTED MEAT

Over the last few decades, we have added antibiotics to meat to kill off the disease our cattle and chickens might have developed. Half of the more than 31 million pounds of antibiotics produced each year in the U.S. are mixed into the feed of cows, pigs and

---

[2] Dr. Neecie Moore, *The Facts about Phytochemicals* (Gharis Publishing Co.: Dallas, Texas, 1996), p. 99.

chickens.[3] Livestock are routinely pumped full of hormones to quickly fatten them for market. Needless to say, an animal's diet impacts its body as much as man's diet impacts his body.

Inspection standards have decreased as contaminants have increased. *The Atlanta Journal-Constitution* interviewed 84 federal poultry inspectors from 27 processing plants in the five states that produce 50 percent of all American chicken. That group reported "seeing millions of chicken each week leaking yellow pus, stained by green feces, contaminated by harmful bacteria, and marred by lung and heart infections and cancerous tumors."[4]

Eating meat or poultry from commercial groceries or restaurants exposes the body to the same diseases found in the source. If you choose to eat meat or poultry, knowing the source is very important. Range-fed meat, wild meat and range-free chickens are a noticeably different breed. Buying animal products from companies such as Coleman Natural (beef and buffalo) or Shelton (chicken and turkey) are worth the slightly higher price. Another source of quality beef is Belle Brook Farms, which provides frozen meat via mail-order. Call 409-560- 9482 for details. The taste is far superior and you can rest in the fact that you are ingesting fewer toxins.

TAINTED DAIRY

In the 40s and 50s many people were getting sick from the consumption of contaminated dairy products. Instead of cleaning up the dairies, legal action was taken to require that all consumer-purchased milk had to be pasteurized. In this process, milk is heated to a high temperature to kill off all bad bacteria. Of course, the heat also kills off anything good in the process. It has been

---

[3] Michael F. Jacobson, Lisa U. Lefferts and Anne Wittee Garland, *Safe Food* (Living Planet Press: Los Angeles, 1991), p. 93.

---

[4] John Robbins, *May All Be Fed* (William Morrow & Co.: New York, 1992), p. 99.

shown in research that taking milk from a cow, pasteurizing it and giving it to her calf will cause the calf to die within six weeks.

Once again, the cattle's diet is questionable. To maximize milk production, cattle are given antibiotics, growth hormones and steroids. During a radio interview, a Canadian dairy farmer told me that the growth hormones approved by the United States Department of Agriculture are illegal in Canada. Canadians know that what is given to a cow affects the milk, which does effect us. When interviewed in the U.S., dairy council members have told me that a cow's diet has no impact on the milk or us. I wonder which comments make more sense?

Detectable amounts of cancer-causing pesticides have been found in pasteurized milk purchased in supermarkets. Unlike bacteria, heat processing does not remove these chemicals.[5] Once again, what goes into the cow has an impact on us.

POLLUTED WATER
Water is crucial for the body, yet pollution has left its mark on this valuable commodity. Roughly 70 percent of the body and 90 percent of the brain is comprised of water. Without water we cannot live for long.

Our water is high in chlorine, fluoride, lead, radon and parasites. This pollution is so widespread that the sale of water filtration systems is a booming business. Yet 70 percent of the contaminants that get into the body from water come from bathing, not from drinking, water. When we consider our daily intake of water through drinking and bathing, we can see that our bodies are being washed in toxins.

POLLUTED ENVIRONMENT
Air pollution is at an all time high. Yet other sources of environmental pollution are just as toxic, just less recognized. Working in

---

[5] David and Anne Frähm, *Healthy Habits* (Piñon Press: Colorado Springs, Colorado, 1993), p. 61.

an office building with closed windows, recycled air, under fluorescent lights and in front of a computer is highly toxic.

Regular fluorescent lights do not contain the full spectrum of light. This light imbalance stresses the body. Full-spectrum fluorescent light bulbs are available for purchase and are helpful for many people.

Computers, as do other electrical appliances, emit electro magnetic fields (EMF's). EMF's are a controversial issue in the health industry. However, imagine being next to a stream in the pure air of the Rocky Mountains. Assuming that you like being outside, would you notice a pleasurable difference in the mountain environment versus that of your city office? The cleaner, outdoor air is partially based on the lack of EMF's. Your body can tell a difference.

With my own health, I had a major relapse in disease symptoms when I began to travel. Airplane travel, hotels and continual eating in restaurants greatly sabotaged my health until I learned how to adjust.

In order to cut costs, airlines recycle airplane air approximately every six minutes. That means you breathe every air-borne germ of every passenger on that flight throughout the entire flight time. In addition, airline air is lower in moisture than any desert. This dryness can lead to dehydration. The inflight consumption of alcohol, coffee and soda pop, which act as diuretics, increases the body's dehydration problem by causing the body to use up its limited source of water.

Formaldehyde is another major environmental contaminant. Formaldehyde is used not only to embalm dead people, it is used in new construction, paint, wallpaper adhesive, fabric, shoulder pads, nail polish and many other manufactured products. When entering shopping malls, the formaldehyde fumes can quickly cause eyes to redden and tear.

Our environment is accosted from all fronts. As we walk, fly, work or play, we are exposed to toxins. We breathe them, touch them and wear them. Our environment is being decorated with toxins more than ever before.

LACK OF ENZYMES

Enzymes are the spark plugs of health. Without enzymes, we are limited in digestion and assimilation of food and supplements. How far would we be able to drive if our car had gas, oil, a key in the ignition, but no spark plugs? Not far! That is exactly how far we can go without enzymes.

Enzymes are manufactured by the body and are found in raw fruits and vegetables. Cooking fruits and vegetables kills enzymes when the cooking temperature exceeds 118 degrees. When we are under stress, our bodies' internal enzyme production is shut down or greatly reduced.

A lack of enzymes has been linked to poor digestion. The abundance of advertisements on television for Zantac, Pepsid AC, Tums and other digestive aids indicates the the dramatic increase of digestive problems in this country. Instead of identifying the source of the indigestion and resolving that problem, we mask the symptoms and wonder why our health further deteriorates.

Poor digestion can manifest with dark circles under the eyes, red cheeks, bloating and gas after meals, allergies, and constipation or diarrhea. These problems do not go away when we take antacids. In fact, the antacids can actually compound the problem. Poor digestion means we are not digesting nor assimilating our food or our supplements. Without digestion and assimilation, we are ripe for all kinds of nutritional deficiencies and dis-ease.

LACK OF FIBER

Fiber is our intestinal broom. It helps clean us out. Without fiber, our colon builds up a mucous-based, false lining. This false lining blocks the colon's ability to eliminate fecal matter, impedes absorption of nutrients from the colon and the release of toxins of the body. This buildup of toxins, fecal matter and malabsorption provides a perfect environment for "bad critters" (i.e., parasites, bacteria, yeast, etc.) to thrive.

Fiber comes from whole grains, fruits, vegetables, psyllium, flax and other natural foods. Highly refined foods (i.e., white bread, refined sugar, processed foods, etc.) are the opposite of more natural fiber-rich foods and are actually the key contributors to this false lining.

REFINED SUGAR

Since 1850, sugar consumption has grown from 12 pounds per year per person to 130 pounds per year per person.[6] A tablespoon of refined sugar can lower the immune system by up to 50 percent for as much as three or four hours. Refined sugar was one of the biggest contributors to my depression. Leading nutritionist, Ann Louise Gittleman says that sugar appears to be the real villain behind our three leading killers — heart disease, cancer and diabetes.[7]

Cancer cells feed on sugar, as do yeast, parasites and bacteria. A diet high in refined sugars does not feed you, it feeds disease. If these consequences are not enough, sugar has also been linked to:

- acne
- adrenal exhaustion
- allergies
- anxiety
- arthritis
- behavior problems
- colitis
- constipation
- diabetes
- fatigue
- eczema
- food cravings
- insomnia
- liver dysfuntion
- mood swings

---

[6] Ann Louise Gittleman, *Get the Sugar Out* (Crown Trade Paperbacks: New York, 1997), p. xiii.

---

[7] ibid, p. xxii.

- PMS
- rheumatism
- tooth decay

DAMAGED FATS

Since the onset of "low fat/no fat" products, the average American has gained eight pounds. Many people now believe that all fats and oils are bad for you. Nothing could be further from the truth!

Essential fatty acids (EFA's) are not even in the same family as greasy French fries, margarine, shortening and vegetable oil. Margarines, shortening and vegetable oils have been hydrogenated, making them only one molecule short of plastic. What do you think your body does with plastic? Not much! It sets, along with other damaged fats, in toxic waste dumps waiting to be cleansed and eliminated.

A shortage of the EFA's can show up as:

- aching joints
- angina
- arthritis
- cardiovascular problems
- constipation
- dry hair and nails
- fatigue
- frequent colds
- high blood pressure
- immune weakness
- indigestion
- mental "fog"
- skin disorders

Without the right oils, the body cannot make waterproof membranes for its cells. All metabolic activity occurs in the watery environment inside cells. The water found inside the cells is different from the water found outside the cells. Each cell is enclosed in a membrane that waterproofs the internal workings from the external ones. This cell membrane is comprised of interlinking oil molecules. Damaged fats compromise health and a lack of EFA's contributes to a loss of cell wall integrity.

CAFFEINE

Caffeine is a stimulant. As such, it impacts the adrenal glands. Over time it can exhaust the adrenals. It also destroys vitamin B, the nerve-building vitamin needed to help us handle stress. Caffeine also acts as a diuretic, removing precious water from the body and brain. Both regular and decaffeinated coffee has oxalic acid, which has been linked to osteoporosis and kidney stones.

INADEQUATE CHEWING

Our digestive system includes our mouth, stomach, small intestine (duodenum, jejunu an ileum) and large intestine (colon). Digestion begins with adequate chewing. Saliva mixes with food in the mouth, breaking it down to enhance overall digestion.

When we "gulp" our foods instead of chewing, we hinder that phase of digestion. This puts additional pressure on the remainder of the digestive system and can lead to indigestion. It certainly impacts halitosis (bad breath).

Drinking large amounts of fluids during a meal dilutes digestive juices and slows digestion. It is best to drink fluids, preferably at-room-temperature water, 20 to 30 minutes prior to or two to three hours following a meal. Without adequate saliva and chewing, food is not completely digested nor assimilated.

STRESS

The most overlooked source of toxins is our daily load of stress. We can eat well, take supplements, exercise, drink water, but still be unhealthy if we have a heavy load of stress. Stress overstimulates the adrenals. The adrenal glands sit on top of the kidneys and produce adrenaline, which is our fight-or-flight hormone. When adrenaline is pumping, cholesterol is elevated, digestion is slowed and elimination is slowed.

Overuse of the adrenals has led to one of the most overlooked, undiagnosed problems in America according to Dr. Steve

Nuggent (president of the American Naturopathic Association) — hypo-adrenia. Hypo-adrenia or adrenal exhaustion can manifest as:

♦ low blood sugar
♦ chronic tiredness
♦ allergies
♦ arthritis
♦ poor stamina
♦ inability to handle stress
♦ muscle weakness
♦ scanty hair and grooved nails
♦ salt and sugar cravings
♦ low body temperature
♦ constipation
♦ depression

Stress can lead to nervous breakdowns, heart attacks, strokes and many other malnutrition-related diseases. Stress is a stalker we often overlook in our pursuit of optimal health.

So, are we toxic? At this point, you are probably wondering if there is anyone who is *not* toxic. The fact is, we all are toxic. The variable is how toxic we are, not if we are toxic. The load of toxins on the human body is at an all-time high. If you are living on planet Earth, you are exposed to these toxic sources on a daily basis, in addition to many more health stumbling blocks.

THE ANSWER

The body deals with toxins through neutralizing, transforming or eliminating them. Various antioxidant nutrients (i.e., vitamins C and E, phytochemicals and some minerals) help neutralize toxins, which cause free-radical damage. This damage breaks down the immune system, making it vulnerable to autoimmune diseases.

Various organs, such as the liver, can transform some toxic substances into harmless elements. These substances are then removed via the blood or bile from the liver. Eventually they are excreted through the urine and fecal matter.

We can also clear some toxins through sweat if the skin is not clogged. Our sinuses expel toxins via the mucous and our skin releases toxins through skin rashes. The body is in constant search of effective ways to slough off toxins.

The problem occurs when our intake of toxins exceeds the body's ability to expel them. This buildup creates major traffic jams inside your body. Today you are an accumulation of all the unloaded toxins you have accumulated since conception. That buildup grows as your toxic load increases. The only variable you face is how this toxic load will manifest — which disease statistic will you become?

Here is where we can help our bodies. Cleansing is a gift you can give your body and your health. Our tour of health must include cleansing because the toxic load we carry has gone beyond acceptable. No longer can the average body neutralize or transform all of the toxins contained within. The next step must be ... cleansing ... if health is a desired goal. If health is not a goal, let sickness and premature death come, unrestrained.

THREE
WHAT IS A CLEANSE?
✦✦✦

Can you image using the same plate to eat dinner tonight that you used for lunch today, yesterday and the day before, without *washing* it? Doesn't that sound offensive? Yet, we rarely think about the fact that leftover food has accumulated inside our bodies. Just as our plates need to be washed, so do the insides of our bodies.

In chapter two, we saw there are a myriad of access points for toxins to enter the body. If a small pebble of sand in a shoe or an eyelash in an eye can irritate, certainly years of accumulated toxins can irritate and damage. So, how do we deal with unwanted substances that enter us via food, air or water? How can we determine what needs to be cleansed, how to cleanse and how efficiently detoxification is being performed within our own bodies? Learning the answers to those questions will help you to understand cleansing, how to do it easily, on a budget and with practical strategies.

DETOXIFICATION DEFINED
The detoxification (or cleansing) process in adults is the major molecule-making activity performed by the body.[1] Most detoxifica-

---

[1] Sidney MacDonald Baker, M.D., *Detoxification and Healing: The Key to Optimal Health* (Keats Publishing, Inc.: New Canaan, Connecticut, 1997), p. 140.

tion occurs during the night between 1:00 a.m. and 3:00 a.m. To understand what is happening inside of the body, let's look at how the body delegates its energy on a normal day.

- ◆ 80% detoxifying
- ◆ 5% immune building
- ◆ 10% thinking
- ◆ 5% maintenance of organs

Cleansing, just as at home, occurs in phases. When we dispose of trash in our home, two phases occur. We prepare the trash by bagging it and then take it in trash cans to the curb for weekly removal. The first phase of removal occurs when the trash is collected. The second phase occurs when the trash is removed.

When our bodies need to remove the "trash," the first phase is to make the unwanted molecules "sticky" or available for removal. These activated molecules can be a mess — just like an uncapped bottle of glue. It is accessible and handy, but it can make a mess if spilled. Just as glue will stick to virtually anything, activated molecules can stick to virtually anything.

As soon as the unwanted toxins are activated, it is important for the trash man to remove the trash. This process is called conjugation or the second phase. Once an activated molecule is attached to a carrier, it becomes deactivated and is flushed out of the body through the blood or bile via the kidneys or intestines.

THE PREVENTION PROCESS

Cleansing also includes preventing the toxins from entering the body. Lifestyle and dietary changes help prevent toxins from entering. Avoiding refined sugar, refined foods (i.e., frozen meals, packaged foods, fast food meals, etc.), white flour, soda pop, caffeine, alcohol, tobacco, drugs and tainted meat and tainted dairy helps minimize the toxic load.

Avoiding environments packed with chemicals also reduces the load. Those environments include new building construction, remodeling, pesticides, sprays and exposure to other chemicals.

Drinking lots of pure water helps flush out toxins. Adding fiber helps brush away toxins collected in the colon. These strategies can help minimize the number of toxins the body has to eliminate. This can help you lessen the load on your cleansing organs thereby supporting them, instead of stressing them.

All foods lean toward being potentially toxic or potentially detoxifying. The following chart points the direction with which foods occur in the terrain of toxicity. This chart is provided in detail in the excellent book, *The Detox Diet* by Elson M. Haas, M.D.

More Congesting ←←← **FOOD** →→→ **Least Congesting**

drugs	sweets	roots	squash	fruits
fried foods	milk	seeds	grains	greens
refined flour	eggs	beans	pasta	herbs
damaged fats	meat	baked goods	nuts	water
			potatoes	

In addition to food and environment, it is important to deal with emotional and spiritual issues to help prevent a buildup of emotional toxicity. (Emotional toxicity was covered in chapter two.) Spiritual vulnerability occurs when a person has no sense of purpose in life. Without a purpose and reason to be alive, or a vital relationship with the Living God, the price to get health is usually too high.

Since most of us do not do everything perfectly, we can benefit from the corrective process of cleansing, as well as the prevention activities. Let's review the cleansing process and its associated benefits.

CLEANSING AND ITS BENEFITS

Cleansing brings many benefits to the body. During or after a cleanse, it is possible for a person to experience improved health, increased energy, fewer symptoms and less fatigue. I always feel better during and after a cleanse. However, when I was highly toxic, some cleanses did cause a time of fatigue.

Some of the benefits to be experienced from cleansing can include:

- clearer skin
- appearance of age reversal
- fewer symptoms
- cleaner body
- organ rest
- weight loss
- improved flexibility
- improved fertility
- less stress
- stable moods
- increased sense of taste
- productivity
- energy
- creativity
- more relaxed
- increased ability to hear God's voice

You might not experience all of these benefits during or after your first cleanse. However, it is possible to experience several of them, especially over time. As I have learned how to do gentle cleansing on a daily basis, as well as stronger cleansing on an as-needed basis, I have found the return well worth the investment.

THE BEST TIME TO CLEANSE

I have found that following trips, holidays and times of excess, I feel better when I cleanse. During times of added stress, I feel better with a simpler intake of food. Seasonally, spring and fall are considered ideal times to cleanse, with spring being the best.

CLEANSING CAUTIONS

If an intense cleanse is started, it is important to work under the supervision of a health care provider. Releasing too many toxins can cause a person to feel sicker. People with cancer and/or saline or silicone implants need to be very careful how they cleanse. In fact, I recommend they *only* cleanse under the supervision of a highly qualified health care provider.

Cleansing should be avoided prior to surgery and four to six weeks following surgery, unless otherwise directed by a health care provider. Pregnant and nursing women should avoid heavy cleansing as it can trigger miscarriages or impact the baby. Mild cleansing can be done, if approved by a health care provider.

When we began our cleansing process while I was quite ill, Forest (my husband) decided to join me. Believing that herbs were only weak little weeds, he decided to step up to the plate and double everything I was doing. Well, these weak little herbs did their job and he began to detox too quickly. He entered into what is called a healing crisis.

HEALING CRISIS AND RETRACING

A healing crisis can occur when we overload the detox pathways with too many toxins; in other words, a "dirty traffic jam" occurs. Too many toxins and too few exits lead to feeling not so good. At this time, a person may experience flu-like symptoms, an increase of the symptoms they are trying to eliminate or extreme fatigue. All of these factors give rise to the benefits of working with a qualified health care provider.

In America we have a commonly accepted belief that the roots of symptoms should be ignored while instant relief to the symptoms is sought. As a result, when we have a symptom such as a cough, fever, cold, headache, rash or diarrhea, we seek a "silver bullet" to give relief. The root of the symptom is never addressed; the root grows, and further health problems develop.

These symptoms are the body's way of communicating that there is an imbalance and that it is trying to remove toxins. When we seek regular relief from these symptoms through medication, we deny the body's miraculous defense — the immune system — from doing its job. This results in a weakened immune system and buildup of toxic waste dumps.

Uncomfortable reactions can occur as you begin to physiologically balance your body chemistry and revitalize your immune system. The longer deficiencies have existed, the more prevalent a response is likely to be. The reactions can appear as: fever, rash or hives, excessive gas, runny nose, headaches, insomnia, increased thirst, weakness, lethargy, loss of appetite, nausea, diarrhea, fever blisters, dry mouth, canker sores, constipation, dizziness, nervousness and various aches and pains. As these reactions occur during cleansing, be assured your body is making positive changes toward an improved state of health.

When we view a symptom as the *problem* instead of the *result* of a problem, we make a major tactical mistake. Continually focusing on symptoms allows a patient to maintain a lifetime of disease and medical treatments; hence, an American health care crisis. If you can recognize these symptoms as correcting crises, it will be easier to accept them as steps on the road to better health. These symptoms are a small price to pay for long-term benefits.

When we view these symptoms as a signal to cleanse, we have the opportunity to allow the immune system to do its job. We support the healing process from within and cleansing can occur.

The key here is to achieve balance. We want to cleanse quickly enough to see results, but not so quickly as to overload the detox highways. When we overload the highways, we create what is known as a healing crisis. During a healing crisis, we may experience more intense healing symptoms than are comfortable. Working with a competent health care provider can help you balance out this process. Doing a more gentle daily cleanse can help eliminate this problem.

The other key in the cleansing process is to recognize the sequence of toxin removal. A good picture of this concept is to view a staircase. Each step represents a level of experience of toxic exposure. As we go down each step, we encounter various toxins or imbalances. Each downward step leads us away from health and into sickness.

In order to go back up the staircase away from sickness toward health, we must reverse the process that caused us to go down. Each step we went down, we must now go up. The way we do that is to cleanse the toxin that entered our body at each step of health deterioration. As we cleanse out the toxins from one level, we can move back up the staircase toward health.

In the world of toxins, this means that the body first cleanses from the inside out; second, the body cleanses from most critical to least critical; and third, the body cleanses the most current toxins first and oldest toxins last. No matter which method of cleansing is utilized, this process of going back up the staircase toward health is called "retracing."

As the body retraces and removes old toxins, it is possible to release heavy metals from the tissue and actually taste them in the mouth. It is also possible to release old chemical exposures and release them through the skin and actually smell the chemical. It is important to understand what is happening so that a person is not unnecessarily alarmed. The releasing of old toxins is the body's way to cleanse itself and bring you health. Instead of fighting them, realize the retraced steps and mild healing crises are bringing you closer to optimal health.

WORDS OF ENCOURAGEMENT

Since I began my adventure to pursue health in 1990, cleansing knowledge, products and information have greatly increased. To-day, it is possible to find quality cleansing products to be used on a daily basis at home. It is possible to find books to help de-mystify and remove fear of the cleansing process for the average consumer.

I have done literally hundreds of cleansing regimes and used many cleansing products. I can truthfully say that my health is bet-ter than ever. I feel better, look better and have fewer health prob-lems than I did 10 years ago. I highly recommend taking the next step to learn how you can clean up your body and experience some of the dramatic improvements that a "clean" bill of health truly provides!

FOUR
HOW TO CLEANSE
✦✦✦

I always recommend that you work with a health care provider prior to starting any cleansing process. For more information on finding a health care provider, check out the information contained in Appendix F.

METHODS OF CLEANSING

There are as many variations to cleansing as there are people alive. Most methods can be divided into four categories:

- ♦ water therapy
- ♦ dietary changes
- ♦ supplemental support
- ♦ additional cleanses

WATER THERAPY

Water therapy covers both internal and external uses of water. The easiest cleanse of all is to ensure that you are drinking enough purified water each day. To determine your recommended water intake, take your body weight and divide by two. This indicates the number of ounces to be consumed each day. For example, if you weigh 150 pounds, the process would be:

150 ÷ 2 = 75 ounces

(8 ounces = 1 cup, therefore 75 ounces = 9 to 10 cups, not glasses, of water.)

DETOX BATHS

Detox baths are an easy, effective and inexpensive method of cleansing. Since up to 70 percent of the contaminants that enter the body via water enter through the skin from bathing or showering, it is very helpful to have a shower filter or house filtration system.

Shower filters can be purchased from your local health food store or Lifestyle for Health. They average from $40 to $120. Whole house systems are more expensive, but they also improve the water in bathing, drinking, cooking, cleaning and laundering. They will also help save on the wear and tear of appliances (i.e., dishwasher, washer, pipes, etc.).

Use one of these methods to bring clean water into the tub for a detox bath. A variety of ingredients can be added to the water for cleansing. (Using an ozonator with your bath helps eliminate parasites. Call LFH for information.) The water should be as hot as the person can stand. The heat and steam increase sweat and open the pores, allowing toxic-sweat to more readily exit the skin.

Should you experience dizziness, headache, exhaustion, fatigue, nausea or weakness at any time during the bath, stop the bath. This is an indication that you are cleansing too quickly, or that your toxic load is too heavy at this time.

Bath Procedure

- ♦ Use a clean tub.
- ♦ Use water as hot as possible that is comfortable.
- ♦ Cover the overflow valve so the water level can be high enough for you to submerge your body up to your neck.
- ♦ Stop the bath if you experience any of the previously mentioned symptoms (wait to stand until you feel strong enough to safely do so).
- ♦ Take a cleansing shower following the bath by using a gentle cleanser and rinse thoroughly.

- In most cases, detox baths can be taken one to three times a week or as needed. (Most health care providers suggest doing a detox bath three times per week, during a cleanse.)
- If tolerated, take extra vitamin C before and after baths.
- Drink eight ounces of pure water before or during the bath.

Types of Baths

Epson Salts. My personal favorite detox bath is with Epson salts. The magnesium content of salts helps relax tired muscles. The sulfur component aids in detoxing. The salts help increase blood supply into the skin and change the pH of the skin surface. The more acid the body is, the easier it is for sickness and disease to occur. A healthy body tends to have a balanced pH level.

Begin with ¼ cup and increase to two to four pounds of salts per bath. I use two to four pounds after each airplane trip, after a day in a TV studio or a day in front of my computer. Yes, with a little swishing, the salts will dissolve in a full tub of water. I find this bath to be quite relaxing and I sleep soundly afterwards.

Apple Cider Vinegar. Vinegar also helps increase blood supply to the skin and change the pH balance. Start with ¼ cup and gradually increase to one cup per bath. I recommend getting raw apple cider vinegar. I never recommend the use of distilled, white vinegar for anything except cleaning windows ... it is never good for you.

Soda. Baking soda creates an alkalinizing bath. This means it will help restore the acid/alkaline balance of the skin. A baking soda bath is very helpful when a person wants to dry weeping, open sores. Use eight ounces of baking soda per bath.

Soda and Salt. An equal combination of baking soda and sea salt can be effective for detoxing from X-ray and radiation exposure. Use equal amounts of soda and non-iodized sea salt, starting with four ounces of each and building to one pound of each.

Ginger Root. Ginger's heating property stimulates the body to sweat. It also helps stimulate and draw toxins to the skin's surface. Use a half inch slice of fresh ginger root (found in produce isle of health food stores and some grocery stores). Place in a pan of water and bring to a boil. Turn off heat and steep for 30 minutes. Remove the ginger piece and pour the liquid into hot bath water.

Herbal Tea. A variety of herbal teas can be used to facilitate detoxing and cleansing chemicals. Some favorites include catnip, peppermint, chamomile, horsetail and yarrow. Use one cup of the brewed tea per tub of water. To make one cup of tea, brew one tablespoon of leaves with one cup of boiling water. Use only one herb at a time. Sensitive people may not do well with herbal baths.

DIETARY CHANGES

Eating a clean diet can be both cleansing and preventive. A clean diet can become a lifestyle of eating and has for our family.

An Example of a Clean Diet

- ◆ Eat organic foods.
- ◆ Eat local, vine-ripened produce.
- ◆ Rotate foods so that allergy introduction is minimized as much as possible. (This is especially true of grains, eggs and yeast foods.)
- ◆ Eat seasonal produce (i.e., during spring, eat foods naturally available in the spring in your locale, etc.).
- ◆ Include a minimum of five servings of fruits and vegetables each day.
- ◆ Use whole grains, not refined grains such as white flour (white flour acts like refined sugar in the body and has no available nutritional content).
- ◆ Avoid aluminum and iron pans. (The aluminum leaches into the food, into the body and is considered toxic and a link to Alzheimer's disease.)
- ◆ Avoid commercial meats, cured meat, refined foods, canned foods, sugar, salt, saturated fats, coffee, alcohol and nicotine. (For further information on each of these foods, please see my book *Food Smart!*)

In addition to eating a clean diet, it is also important to know your metabolic profile. In my book *Revised Meals in 30 Minutes*, I provide the reader with a personalized profile and understanding of how to determine whether they are a fast, slow or balanced burner. Knowing your own profile allows you to blend proteins, carbohydrates and fats in exactly the right proportion for your body. This balanced fuel mix provides more energy and helps balance weight, along with many other benefits. From a cleansing perspective, it allows for maximum energy so that the body actually has the energy it needs to cleanse.

Fasting
Some people choose to fast in order to cleanse. Never attempt a long-term fast (more than three days) without medical supervision. Fasting can help the body to heal and to resist infections, dis-eases and toxins. Fasting is occurring when we find ourselves not wanting food when we are sick. This is a natural response and should be honored.

During sensible fasting, the body produces new healthy cells to replace tired, toxic cells. Many people opt for a liquid-only day each week, which brings 52 days of cleansing to the body each year. Other people choose to do three day fasts each month, which gives the body 36 days of fasting each year.

The toxins stored in our fat cells and organs are rapidly released during a fast. If a person is highly toxic, has cancer or silicon/saline implants, fasting can release too many toxins at one time. It is critical with any fast to drink at least eight to ten glasses (not just cups) of liquid each day.

Green powders, such as KyoGreen, added to vegetable juice or water is an excellent rejuvenating drink to do two to three times per day while fasting. In addition to green drinks, a drink made with equal parts (approximately one tablespoon) pure maple syrup and cider vinegar to one cup of warm water is helpful. For people with candida (overgrowth of yeast) the syrup and vinegar can be replaced with freshly squeezed lemon juice. The syrup/vinegar drink helps restore internal pH balance.

To eliminate trauma and retain benefits, break a fast carefully. Eat a light, first meal and chew thoroughly. A sample of an optimal fast breaking menu includes:

1st day	fresh fruit in a.m.
	vegetable salad in p.m.
2nd day	fresh fruit in a.m.
	vegetable salad in p.m.
	vegetable soup for dinner
3rd day	more fruit in a.m.
	vegetable salad in p.m.
	nuts (if digested), fermented dairy (if tolerated)
	or baked potato
4th day	start back on mild food

Fasting can be water only, liquids only, or a Daniel's fast, which is primarily vegetables. In most cases, supplements are not taken during a one to three day fast. However, supplements are usually necessary to help replace the body's depleted nutrient stores. Although vitamins and minerals can interfere with cleansing, herbs can help the cleansing process.

SUPPLEMENTAL SUPPORT

Cleansing requires a large amount of energy. Various supplements are helpful to increase available energy and nutrients to facilitate the body's cleansing. Some nutrients are critical for necessary chemical reactions to occur in the cleansing process.

The following supplemental support helps in either the cleansing phase and/or the building phase.

- ◆ fiber
- ◆ probiotics
- ◆ glyconutrition
- ◆ EFA's
- ◆ enzymes
- ◆ daily vitamins
- ◆ macro and trace minerals
- ◆ vitamin E
- ◆ antioxidants

- amino acids
- aloe vera

Fiber

Fiber provides the bulk to cleanse the colon. Examples of excellent fiber includes pysllium seed husk, flaxseed, carrageenan, oats and whole grains. Some of these foods can be obtained in a daily diet or daily fiber supplement. Some psyllium drinks also contain bentonite. Research has shown the bentonite can contain toxic levels of aluminum. We have personally discontinued fiber drinks or cleanses containing bentonite. When taking fiber as a supplement, it is imperative to drink the full amount of water your body needs. (See formula under water therapy in this chapter.)

Probiotics

Most of us have heard of antibiotics. Their healthier counterparts are called probiotics. Maintaining a balance between the harmful "critters" and the good "critters" enhances the body's production of natural antibodies. Hypersensitivity and autoimmune diseases can be increased due to a lack of good bacteria in the colon.

The body needs approximately three pounds of good "critters." Stress, prescription antibiotics and meat and dairy products containing antibiotics rob the body of these good "critters." When the GI (gastrointestinal) tract's membranes are compromised from a lack of good bacteria, the condition called "leaky gut" can occur. With leaky gut, large molecules of toxins cross the intestinal wall and can lead to autoimmune diseases (i.e. cancer, multiple sclerosis, fibromyaliga, arthritis, etc.) or inflammation of muscles and joints. These large molecules are able to pass through the intestinal wall, because the wall's integrity has been compromised from toxins, increased numbers of "critters" and a lack of water.

Lactobacilli are one of the five major groups of intestinal bacteria. Lactobacillus refers to the bacteria that produce lactic acid. Examples of latobacilli include acidophilus, planetarium, rhamosus and casei. Lactobacilli are effective against 25 strains of bad bacteria, including staphylococcus, salmonella and streptococcus.

Another category of good intestinal bacteria is called bifidobacteria. They comprise about 25 percent of the beneficial intestinal bacteria. The increased growth of bifidobacteria can help lower blood pressure, cholesterol and detoxify carcinogens in the intestines. An example of bifidobacterium is bifidum.

Glyconutrition
Glyconutrition is the nutrition coming from glycoproteins that promote cellular communication. Glycoproteins are molecules found on the surface of cells. They are constructed from glyco (sugar from carbohydrates) and protein, and are responsible for cell to cell communication (a system that is similar to cell phones or the Internet). The body breaks down plant carbohydrates, restructures them into small sugars, then uses those sugars to build the glycoproteins required for your "cell phones" to work.

The glyco sugars are not like refined table sugar. They are monosaccharides, which are single sugars the body needs as raw materials to build glycoproteins. Our bodies require eight monosaccharides in order to build glycoproteins and have cells clearly communicating.

Only two of these essential sugars are found in classical nutritional textbooks, the other six are omitted due to the fact that they are uncommon in today's diet. These other six sugars must be either synthesized by the body or obtained from dietary supplements. They are essential in the cleansing and building process so that the body's command centers (cell phones) can function. Without them the body can misuse or even fail to use incoming nutrients and supplements.

One of the key sugars in the field of glyconutrition is the sugar mannose. Mannose is the active component of the aloe vera plant, which is well known for its healing properties. Mannose is one of the eight sugars known to promote cleansing, cellular communication and rebuilding. Ambrotose™ is a glyconutritional supplement containing mannose and the seven other necessary monosaccharides. More information on this product can be found in Appendix A.

EFA's

Essential fatty acids are called essential because your body does not manufacture them. They must come through diet and supplementation. EFA's are the building blocks of healthful fats that the body needs to function and are key structural components of cell membranes and of intracellular structure. They are also a major source of energy.

Enzymes

Enzymes are the small proteins that cause chemical reactions in the cells and also help build glycoproteins. Enzymes require adequate supplies of monosaccharides (sugars) to form glycoproteins and accelerate bodily reactions that would otherwise be too slow. They help the body form nerve impulses to regulate hormones. Enzymes enable our body to renew old cells, metabolize nutrients into building blocks for energy, and remove waste products and toxins. Enzymes are essential to the function of vitamins and minerals.

Metabolic enzymes are found in the body. About 5,000 metabolic enzymes operate the body's internal chemistry. One type of metabolic enzyme, antioxidant enzymes, converts free radicals (the precursors of aging process and cancer) into water and oxygen, which helps detox the body.

Food enzymes, found in raw foods, help in the digestion and assimilation process. Those enzymes include:

- ♦ amylase (starch digestion)
- ♦ protease (protein digestion)
- ♦ lipase (fat digestion)
- ♦ cellulose (fiber digestion)
- ♦ saccharase (sugar digestion)
- ♦ lactase (milk sugar digestion)

Digestive enzymes from food work in the stomach. Digestive enzymes from the pancreas work in the small intestine. Enzyme supplementation is often helpful, especially when the diet is low in raw fruits and vegetables, during times of stress and/or during times of cleansing.

Daily Vitamin and Mineral Support

Vitamins and minerals, either from the diet or supplements, are essential in the chemical reactions which happen in the detoxification process. Supplementation through a daily vitamin and mineral is a widely accepted method of ensuring adequate vitamin and mineral levels. The key is to ensure that the daily vitamin/supplement is balanced with each individual's unique requirements. Research indicates that although all of us need every vitamin and mineral, the necessary quantity of each can vary dramatically from one person to another.

Knowing your metabolic profile, specific food needs (fat, protein and carbohydrate balance), along with the appropriate formula of vitamins and minerals for you can optimize the effectiveness of your cleanse. Metabolic profiling is covered extensively in my book, *Revised Meals in 30 Minutes.*

Macro and Trace Minerals

Every second of every day your body relies on trace minerals in an ionic form to conduct and generate billions of tiny electrical impulses. (Ionic means the minerals are in a form that does not require digestion — they go straight to the cells.) Without these impulses, not a single muscle would be able to function. Your brain would fail to function and the cells would not be able to use osmosis to balance water pressure and absorb nutrients. In fact, "many vital body processes depend on the movement of ions across cell membranes." [1]

Minerals should be ionic in order for the body to more easily absorb and transfer them into the small intestine. Minerals are absorbed in their ionic form as a liquid solution and have either a positive or negative charge. Balanced ionic minerals help with biochemical communication throughout the body.

---

[1] American Medical Association, *The American Medical Association's Encyclopedia of Medicine*, ed. Charle b. Clayman. (Random House: New York, 1989), p. 605.

Vitamin E

Vitamin E is the most important antioxidant found in the body. It enhances various parts of the detox process and helps increase the oxygenation process. It is important when a person has been exposed to smog, smoking, sun or X-rays, which lead to cellular deterioration. Vitamin E deficiency increases vulnerability to lung damage caused by ozone.

Vitamin E can be found in green leafy vegetables, whole grains, milk fat, butter, egg yolks, nuts and supplements. It is found in large amounts in the brain, pituitary gland and adrenal glands. Always begin vitamin E supplements in small amounts.

Appendix A gives you names of products we have found effective and affordable in reaching cleansing and supplement goals.

ADDITIONAL CLEANSING METHODS

Skin Brushing

The skin eliminates more cellular waste than the colon and kidneys combined. Brushing the skin when it is dry helps this elimination process. It also helps stimulate the lymph system, which carries nutrients to the cells and helps eliminate toxins from the cells.

Natural bristle skin brushes can be purchased in health food and department stores or from Lifestyle for Health. They come in medium and firm bristle strengths. To start, medium is preferred.

Two pairs of ducts are key for lymph drainage. One pair is located by the collar bone. The other set is located in the groin folds. Hand massaging each set of ducts prior to skin brushing is helpful for drainage. To brush the skin, use small circular motions starting close to the ducts and moving out toward the extremities. From the waist up, brush toward the upper ducts. From the waist down, brush toward the groin ducts. Brushing should take three to five minutes before each shower.

Organ Cleansing

The two major organs that detox the body are the liver and colon. During times of stress and/or toxic overload, it can be helpful to do an intense cleanse of the liver and colon. This type of cleansing is best done under the care of a health care provider.

More gentle dietary and herbal support of the liver and colon can be done at anytime. Those supports include the use of:

♦ dandelion, milk thistle or fennel herbal supplements (Remedies with these herbs can be found in your local health food store. Follow directions on bottles.)
♦ avoiding margarine and shortening (These foods negatively impact both the colon and liver.)
♦ cold-pressed oils in small amounts (These are healthier oils to be used in cooking.)
♦ light, easy to digest foods
♦ green, slightly bitter vegetables For example, endive, collards and dandelion help activate the bile flow, which helps cleanse the liver.
♦ allowing 12 hours between the evening and morning meals to give the colon a chance to process food in a more efficient manner
♦ lemon water that can be made by squeezing half of a lemon into a quart of purified water (This helps restore pH balance and cleanse the liver.)

Cleansing of the liver can also include liver massage. Lying flat on the back, use your fingertips and gently massage the liver area. The liver can be found by placing your right hand at the base of your right rib cage. Massage in a clockwise circular motion for three to five minutes at a time, two to three times per day.

Coffee Enemas
Coffee enemas are considered by many to be one of the best liver cleansers. A coffee enema is a low-volume cleanse that helps detox in many ways. It helps to speed up the bowel's emptying process, which makes the detox process occur more quickly. It also helps the liver empty toxins found in the bile ducts. Coffee enemas do not wash out minerals and electrolytes, which are absorbed higher in the bowel. Do not do coffee enemas if gallstones are present.

People sensitive to coffee are often reluctant to try coffee enemas. Since the coffee stays in the sigmoid colon and the caffeine only goes into the liver circulatory system, it is usually safe to use. Consult with your health care provider and use organic coffee. Not knowing the decaf process, I do not recommend using decaf coffee.

To do a coffee enema, heat one quart of purified water to a boil. Add two flat tablespoons of organic coffee and boil for five minutes. Turn off heat. Cool to a lukewarm temperature. Strain out the coffee grounds.

Place the strained coffee liquid into an enema bag. Be sure the tubing is clamped shut. Hang the enema bag at waist level. Hanging the bag too high will force the fluid too high into the intestine. Lie on a covered floor. Insert the enema nozzle, which may be lubricated if needed. Release the clamp and let about half of the coffee flow in. If possible, retain the enema for 10 minutes. After that time period (or sooner, if needed), reclamp the tube, remove the nozzle and empty the bowels into the toilet. Repeat process with remaining half of enema.

Liver/Gallbladder Flush
The bile produced by the liver is stored in the gallbladder. When the liver secretes too much cholesterol or the bile becomes too highly concentrated in the gallbladder, then gallstones form. The gallbladder favors a diet higher in protein and lower in refined carbohydrates. B-vitamin complex, lecithin and vitamin E help the gallbladder.

To flush the liver and gallbladder, cleanse the bowels via fasting, colemas or enemas. This should occur for three to five days prior to the flush. Fast two days prior to the flush. Always consult a health care provider prior to cleansing.

On the first day of the flush, drink one to two glasses of organic apple juice (Mountain Sun is my favorite) every two hours. Do not eat during that day. Follow the same process on the second day. At bedtime drink four ounces of olive oil (preferably organic, expeller pressed) followed with a ½ cup of orange or lemon juice chaser. Usually this flush starts to work the second day. Small stones and/or green mud should be eliminated in the fecal matter.

Colon Cleansing
The colon often becomes the breeding ground for the bad "critters." It can also develop a false lining from eating the Standard American Diet (SAD), which retards the absorption of nutrients. Probiotics help to recolonize the colon with good bacteria.

Additional colon cleansing can be done through colemas or colonics. These methods are somewhat controversial. For a thorough discussion of these methods, I recommend Dr. Jacqueline Krohn's book *The Whole Way to Natural Detoxification* (Hartley & Marks Publishers, 1996). I personally have done many colemas and have found them to be helpful in cleansing my colon.

Deep Breathing
Breathing is the only function of the body that can be performed both consciously and unconsciously. Many health problems are impacted by shallow breathing. Many emotions can be soothed with slow, deep, regular breathing.

To breathe deeply, sit in a chair with both feet on the ground or stand with both feet equally balanced on the ground. Relax the shoulders. Breathe in deeply through the nose. When you breathe deeply, the shoulders do not move up, instead the diaphragm or chest moves out. Breathe in deeply to the count of three, hold the breath for a count of three, then slowly release the breath to the count of three. Doing this exercise throughout the day brings additional oxygen into the body and helps release stress.

Regularly service any furnace, humidifier or air conditioner in your home and working environment. Keeping these machines clean and keeping the filters changed improves the quality of the air you are breathing. You may also want to have your air ducts professionally cleaned.

The best air is found outside, when it is free of pollution. Taking early morning walks and breathing deeply is good for cleansing and healing. The air we exhale removes some toxins, so breathe deeply. Twenty minutes of fresh air and sunshine is an excellent cleanser and rejuvenator.

Exercise

Be sure to check with your health care provider before starting any new exercise program.

Exercise helps remove toxins as much as some internal cleansers. Exercise strengthens the heart muscle and improves blood circulation. The better our circulation, the better our delivery system for bringing nutrition to the cells and removing toxins. Regular exercise improves metabolism, the rate with which we burn calories for energy. Exercise also stimulates digestion and improves elimination, all of which are important for cleansing.

Research indicates that exercise raises the level of the HDL (good) cholesterol while lowering the LDL (bad) cholesterol levels. Blood pressure can be lowered through exercise. Weight-bearing exercise (which means exercises utilizing weight) builds strong bones by helping them to retain calcium, thereby helping preven osteoporosis.

Exercise stimulates the pituitary gland, which releases endorphins. Endorphins have a tranquilizing affect upon us and are released about 30 minutes after aerobic exercise. Stress can often be minimized as a result of a release of endorphins.

SUMMARY

There are many options for the cleansing process to occur in your body and life. The key is to not be overwhelmed with the variety. Instead, identify one or two steps that you can successfully and consistently implement. Usually the easier the cleanse, the easier for you and the more your confidence is built. The more consistent the application, the easier it becomes to make cleansing a part of your regular lifestyle.

I have done each of these cleanses many times. I know people who do some of the cleanses and not all of the cleanses. I also know people who have done none of these cleanses and these people tend to have many more health "challenges." Start where you are and do what you can. If you can only do a detox bath once a month, you are at least moving in the right direction.

Because cleansing can be overwhelming, I am very excited about the MannaCleanse™ product produced by Mannatech™. MannaCleanse was designed by industry experts Ann Louise Gittleman, Chris Moore and Dan McAnalley. It is discussed in Appendix A, is a caplet and can be taken every day.

The real key to cleansing is to ... start! Whether you do a simple, effective cleanse like MannaCleanse, or you add other cleansing processes to MannaCleanse, just start! No cleanse is effective when it is not implemented.

FIVE
CLEANSING ᴬᴺᴰ CHILDREN
✦✦✦

I always recommend that you work with a qualified health care provider any time you are considering starting a cleanse with a child.

A fetus, newborn and infant are extremely vulnerable to toxins. Their cells are rapidly dividing, their metabolic rate is high and their immune system is immature. The first trimester of pregnancy is the most vulnerable time during pregnancy. The surface area covered by a baby's skin is three times larger than an adult's, relative to their corresponding weights. All of this impacts a child's susceptibility to toxins.

PRIMARY TOXINS
The primary toxic exposures that impact children include:

- ✦ air
- ✦ foods and plants
- ✦ metals
- ✦ organisms
- ✦ pesticides
- ✦ radiation
- ✦ solvents
- ✦ water

AIR

Young children have a more rapid respiratory rate and higher metabolic rate then adults and are therefore more sensitive to air pollution. Asthma impacts more than three million children in the United States alone. It is now the leading cause of children missing school.

Asthmatic wheezing can be antagonized by perfume, fireplace smoke and cigarette smoke. Children exposed to cigarette smoke have a 50% higher rate of respiratory infection. Babies born to parents who smoke are more likely to die of SIDS (sudden infant death syndrome).

To decrease air allergens, consider not using carpet in bedrooms. Keep pets out of bedrooms. Frequently wash all stuffed animals, curtains, bedspreads and other fabric items.

FOODS AND PLANTS

Breast-fed children tend to have fewer allergies to food. Breast milk has natural antibodies that strengthen a baby's immune system. Children are more vulnerable to food poisoning, especially if they have a weakened immune system. Keep children away from toxic household plants, sprayed lawns and flowers. The sprays used on yards can impact a child through the air they breathe when outside in the yard or when they play in the lawn. This is true for all children.

Because of their size, children are more sensitive to pesticides and chemical residue in food. Many nutritionists recommend organic produce to children for that reason. The fewer the chemicals used in food eaten by a child, the more opportunity the child's immune system is given to develop.

METALS

Lead poisoning is the most common source of metal poisoning in children. Lead impacts the central nervous system. Children are exposed to lead from the air, food and water they are given. A nutritious diet helps a child absorb, retain and store less of this toxic, heavy metal.

Everybody is exposed to lead in this manner. The difference in the results is the strength of the body to eliminate the lead. This is based on the strength of the immune system and the openness of the detox pathways. Children tend to be more vulnerable. Knowing this, parents need to provide clean air, healthy food and purified water to children. My book *Kid Smart!* gives many options for children at different age levels.

ORGANISMS

Children are often exposed to bacteria, parasites and viruses. Homeopathics are well tolerated by infants and children as a means of treatment of these bad "critters." Steam inhalation can help breathing during viral infections.

A homeopathic remedy for a symptom is a microdilution or microdose of the very same plant, mineral or chemical substance that in its original concentration will bring on an illness. For more information on homeopathics, I recommend *Optimal Wellness* by Ralph Golan, M.D.

Hydrogen peroxide can be used to help alleviate skin and/or nail fungal infections.

PESTICIDES

Keeping a home as pest-free as possible is good. However, non-toxic pest control is critical with children. Organic gardening both in your own yard and with purchased produce greatly reduces a child's exposure to pesticides. The Environmental Working Group states that the average child receives up to 35 percent of his or her entire lifetime dose of carcinogenic pesticides by the age of five.[1] If the child is in a weakened health state, this could mean that an occurrence of cancer can occur earlier.

---

[1] Jacqueline Krohn, M.D., *The Whole Way to Natural Detoxification* (Hartley & Marks: Point Roberts, Washington, 1996), p. 191.

RADIATION

Infants and children should not be exposed to the sun without protection. Sunscreens should not be used until at least six months of age, and then they should be nontoxic. The best sun screen is light-weight cotton clothing and a hat.

Children should not be exposed to electric blankets. All electrical items emit EMF (electrical magnetic frequencies). Although this subject is somewhat controversial, most natural health care providers suggest limiting a child's exposure to EMF's.

SOLVENTS

Children are much more sensitive to solvents than are adults. When cleaning or doing laundry, use nontoxic products. Always keep solvents out of the reach of small children. Never place them in a familiar container (i.e., water bottle) which could cause a child to drink them unknowingly.

Freshly decorated nurseries can increase toxicity. New homes, mobile homes and recently decorated homes are highly toxic for children as well as adults. Many people totally overlook the potential side effects of these toxic exposures to children. In the next chapter, we address resources to help reduce the impact of these toxins.

If a child swallows a solvent, do not induce vomiting. Call your poison control center immediately for advice.

WATER

Children should only drink purified water. If traveling, use bottled water. Children dehydrate easily, especially if they have low body weight. Dehydrated children will cry without tears, have a dry mouth and have decreased urination.

CLEANSING METHODS

The more a parent can keep a child away from toxins, the less cleansing is needed. Homeopathic remedies do work well with children. Even if a child spits out a homeopathic remedy, he has still received a small dose. Detox baths (Epson salts, apple cider vinegar and plain water) work well for children. Sauna can even be helpful. Be sure to closely monitor time and temperature of baths.

Organ cleansing and enemas should *NOT* be used with children. Grated flaxseed can be added to drinks to help with constipation. Total fasting should not be done with small children. Older children (those over the age of 10) can usually handle fruit and vegetable cleanses.

Although herbs are usually safe for children, they need to be monitored. Liquid tincture should always be diluted before given to children. Many of the liquid tinctures can be rubbed into the skin of the abdomen instead of taken orally.

Bodywork, such as massage, chiropractic and reflexology is usually quite safe and enjoyable to children. Exercise is key for overall development and internal balancing.

Keeping a child free from toxins is much easier than cleansing. For more information on cleansing and your child, seek the advice of your health care provider.

RECOMMENDATIONS
AND
RESOURCES

(A LITTLE R & R)
✦✦✦

RECOMMENDATIONS
ᴬɴᴅ RESOURCES
♦♦♦

The following product recommendations have not been solicited or paid for. I am not a paid spokesperson for any of the companies listed here.

EVALUATION PROCESS

In order for Lifestyle for Health or me to recommend a product, we first go through an extensive evaluation process. We meet with the president or owner of the company to determine the integrity and mission of the company. We then meet with formulators to determine the quality of design, quality of ingredients and the integrity of the formulation. If at all possible, the processing plant is toured to determine the quality control standards and processing methods used. We check the reputation of the company within the health care and supplement industry. Next, our family tries the product. We also recommend the product to people with specific health problems to evaluate their success.

Based on the effectiveness and results of all of these tests and on the price of the product, we make an evaluation as to whether or not we can wholeheartedly recommend the product. No decision is ever based solely on sales or marketing literature. The following products and services have all been evaluated by using this process. My family and I use — or have used — all of these products and services.

Our recommendations have been categorized in the following manner:

Appendix A: Cleansing and Supplement Products
Appendix B: Cleansing Equipment
Appendix C: Food and Supplement Manufacturers
Appendix D: Recommended Reading and Listening Material
Appendix E: Children's Resources
Appendix F: Health Care Providers

APPENDIX A
CLEANSING AND
SUPPLEMENT PRODUCTS
✦✦✦

The following products were mentioned in the cleanse chapter. The products are listed here with recommended sources. Any Lifestyle for Health product can be purchased by using the attached order form or by calling 303-794-4477.

CLEANSER
My favorite is a cleanse by Mannatech™ called MannaCleanse™. It contains six kinds of fibers, six live probiotics, six flora growth promoters (including Ambrotose™, which has the glyconutrients for cellular communication), six essential oils, six EFA's and six enzymes. Mannatech products can be purchased from a local Mannatech distributor or from Lifestyle for Health.

FIBER
703 Inner Cleanse and Natures Cleanse Package is a combination fiber and enzyme support cleanse for intense cleanses. The 703 Cleanse can be purchased from Lifestyle for Health. Freshly ground flaxseed (found in your local health food store) is an excellent, inexpensive source of dietary fiber.

PROBIOTICS
We use and recommend Infinity Total Flora for a good probiotic. Total Flora contains several different strains of the good bacteria.

Kyolic makes an excellent acidophilus, which can be found in your local health food store. Probiotics are also found in the Manna-Cleanse product. Both MannaCleanse and Total Flora can be purchased from Lifestyle for Health.

GLYCONUTRITIONALS
As of this time Mannatech has the composition of matter patent on the combination of all monosaccharides in the form of Ambrotose. I recommend the use of glyconutritionals to restore cellular communication. Ambrotose can be found in the MannaCleanse product, as well as other Mannatech products and can be purchased from Lifestyle for Health.

ESSENTIAL FATTY ACIDS
The best source of EFA's is a high lignan, organic flaxseed oil. My preference for flaxseed oil is Barlean's. It has superior taste, is organic and comes in both capsule and oil forms. EFA's are also found in the MannaCleanse product. Barlean's products can be found in your local health food store or from Lifestyle for Health. Freshly ground flaxseed (found in your local health food store) is an excellent, inexpensive source of EFA's.

ENZYMES
My favorite dietary enzyme product is called Digest-A-Meal from Infinity. Kyolic also makes a good enzyme, which can be found in your local health food store. Enzymes are in the MannaCleanse product. Both MannaCleanse and Digest-A-Meal can be purchased from Lifestyle for Health.

DAILY VITAMINS
There are many vitamins on the market today — some are effective,some are not. The key is to purchase whole food supplements, not synthetic ones. (For more information on this subject, I recommend the book *The Real Truth About Vitamins and Antioxidants* by Judith A. DeCava.) Whole food vitamins will contain lower dosages than synthetic but we believe they are more effective.

The next step beyond whole food is to get the vitamin customized to an individual's metabolic process. The Profile Vitamins by Mannatech match a slow, fast and balanced burner's metabolic requirements. Profile Vitamins and *The Real Truth About Vitamins and Antioxidants* book can be purchased from Lifestyle for Health.

MACRO AND TRACE MINERALS

Most daily vitamins include the macro minerals. For ionic trace minerals, I recommend ConcenTrace Minerals Drops by Trace Minerals. They are in a liquid, ionic form and are easy to assimilate for children or adults. Trace Mineral products can be found in your local health food store or ordered from Lifestyle for Health.

VITAMIN E

Vitamin E can be purchased from several network marketing companies (i.e., Shaklee, Amway, etc.), health food stores and mail order catalogs. Look for natural sources versus synthetic sources.

ANTIOXIDANTS

Antioxidants can be found as individual products (i.e., greens powders) or in phytochemical supplements. Our favorite greens powder is KyoGreen from Kyolic, which can be found in your local health food store or from Lifestyle for Health.

PHYTOCHEMICALS

Our favorite phytochemical products are PhytoBears (gummy bear form without refined sugar or food coloring) and Phyt-Aloe (capsule form) from Mannatech, which can be purchased from Lifestyle for Health.

ALOE VERA

Aloe vera is known for its healing properties. Manapol™ is the patented name for the mannose molecule that is the active ingredient found in the aloe plant. Manapol can be found in Ambrotose in Mannatech products. Mannatech products can be purchased directly from Lifestyle for Health.

Lifestyle for Health
P.O. Box 3871
Littleton, CO 80161
Phone 303-794-4477
Fax 303-794-1449
E-mail lfhealth@lfhealth.com
www.lfhealth.com

APPENDIX B
CLEANSING EQUIPMENT
♦♦♦

The following equipment has been mentioned throughout this book as being helpful for cleansing. This resource list is not meant to be exhaustive of all possible sources, however, I do recommend these particular sources.

AIR FILTERS

The air filter we use was purchased from Sears, provides negative ions and was under $100. Other quality air filters can be purchased from the Allergy Resource Group.

Allergy Free
1502 Pine Drive
Dickinson, TX 77539
800-ALLERGY

To further cleanse the environment, I recommend a zeolite rock sold by Natural NonScents. (It is effective at removing chemicals, electro magnetic fields and odors. For more information on how this product works, call Natural NonScents.)

Natural NonScents
303-232-2459

COLEMA BOARDS

The colema boards can be purchased from Jubilee-He Restoreth.

Jubilee-He Restoreth
303-805-1618

ENEMA BAGS

The Fleet enema bag is good for enemas and can be found in drug stores such as Walgreens, Payless and in some grocery stores.

HOUSEHOLD CLEANERS

Many excellent companies provide toxin-free household cleaners. These companies include Shaklee, Amway and Ecover.

LAUNDRY PRODUCTS

Many excellent companies provide toxicless laundry products. These companies include Shaklee, Amway and Ecover. I never recommend the use of dryer sheets, as they can aggravate skin problems due to the perfumes and chemicals.

LIVER PACKS

Caster oil can be used for liver packs. Caster oil can be purchased in pharmacies and health food or grocery stores. The best source for organic, expeller pressed caster oil is the Heritage Store.

Heritage Store
800-862-2923

REBOUNDER

Rebounders can be found in your local discount stores such as Walmart. The best type of rebounder that I have found is from Needak™.

Needak Manufacturing
PO Box 776
O'Neill, NE 68763
800-232-5762

SHOWER HEADS

There are many shower heads on the market today. A good brand is Tap Dance, which can be found in health food stores or purchased from Lifestyle from Health.

WATER FILTERS

We have chosen a three-stage, reverse osmosis water filtration system from Shaklee called BestWater. To find the most recent ratings, check the most recent issue of *Consumer Report* magazine covering this topic.

For bottled water I recommend Sports Water by Alacer, Calistoga and Indian Peaks, all of which can be found in all health food stores and some grocery stores.

Lifestyle for Health
P.O. Box 3871
Littleton, CO 80161
Phone 303-794-4477
Fax 303-794-1449
E-mail lfhealth@lfhealth.com
www.lfhealth.com

APPENDIX C
FOOD AND SUPPLEMENT MANUFACTURERS
✦✦✦

The following food and supplement brands have been mentioned throughout this book. I recommend these brands because of their overall commitment to quality and integrity.

FOOD MANUFACTURERS

ALTA DENA

Alta Dena has a great line of quality dairy products, from fresh milk to kefir, yogurt, ice cream and others. They are committed to producing milk products without using bovine growth hormones. Dairy products without this hormone are much safer for you and your family. Alta Dena's quality and integrity are excellent.

> Alta Dena Certified Dairy
> 17637 Valley Boulevard
> City of Industry, CA 91744-5731
> Phone: 818-964-6401
> Fax: 818-965-1960

BARBARA'S BAKERY

Barbara's Bakery provides quality, nutritious foods, from chips, pretzels and cookies to cereals, granola bars, bread sticks and crackers. Their food is tasty and very reasonably priced. Many low-fat and no-fat foods are available.

Barbara's Bakery, Inc.
3900 Cypress Drive
Petaluma, CA 94954
Phone: 707-765-2273

CASCADIAN FARM

Cascadian Farm provides a wealth of excellent products. Many of their products are organic, from their frozen fruits and vegetables to their jams, jellies, preserves, sorbets, pickles and relishes. They have great "popsicles" made with organic milk and unrefined sugar. They have Kosher foods.

Cascadian Farm
P.O. Box 568
Concrete, WA 98237
Phone: 206-855-0100
Fax: 206-855-0444

COLEMAN NATURAL MEATS

Coleman Natural Meats come from cattle that are totally natural and raised without hormones or steroids. The flavor is excellent, beyond comparison with other commercially available meats. They provide beef and other meats.

Coleman Natural Meats Inc.
5140 Race Court #4
Denver, CO 80127
Phone: 303-297-9393
Fax: 303-297-0426

FRONTIER HERBS

Frontier provides fresh herbs in both bulk and packaged forms. They also produce organic coffees. This company is committed to quality and integrity.

Frontier Cooperatives Herbs
1 Frontier Road
P.O. Box 299
Norway, IA 52318
Phone: 800-669-3275

HORIZON

Horizon is a supplier of dairy products that are all organic. Their products are cow, and not goat, based. They carry a full line of milk, cheese and yogurt.

Horizon
Boulder, CO 80301

LUNDBERG

Lundberg produces organic and premium brown-rice products. They also have rice blends, brown-rice cakes, flours, cereals and pilafs. Their brown-rice syrup is an excellent sugar replacement that many diabetics can use. Their brown-rice pudding mixes are excellent, as are their one-step chili mixes.

Lundberg Family Farms
P.O. Box 369
Richvale, CA 95974
Phone: 916-882-4551

MORI NU

Mori Nu has the best silken tofu (a smooth tofu with the texture of sour cream, without the cholesterol). It works the best with many of my recipes. It comes in aseptic packaging for longer shelf life. Their "lite" tofu has the least fat of any tofu on the market.

Mori Nu
2050 West 190th, #110
Torrance, CA 90504
Phone: 800-NOW TOFU
Fax: 310-787-2727

MOUNTAIN SUN

Mountain Sun is committed to organic products. They provide great organic and natural food juices under the labels of Mountain Sun and Apple Hill. Their flavors and varieties are superb.

Mountain Sun
18390 Highway 145
Dolores, CO 81323
Phone: 303-882-2283
Fax: 303-882-2270

MUIR GLEN

Muir Glen tomato products are by far my favorite. These organically grown tomato products are packaged in enamel lined cans, which produces a superior taste and product. Their products range from chunky sauces to paste to whole tomatoes. Throw away those tinny-tasting tomatoes and try Muir Glen.

Muir Glen
424 North 7th Street
Sacramento, CA 95814
Phone: 800-832-6345
Fax: 916-557-0903

PAMELA'S PRODUCTS

Pamela's Products produces our favorite cookies. Many of their cookies are wheat-free, sugar-free and some are dairy-free. A line of biscotti cookies has been added to the regular line.

Pamela's Products
156 Utah Avenue
South San Francisco, CA 94080
Phone: 415-952-4546

SAN-J

San-J has great sauces for stir-fries and marinades. Their tamari has an excellent flavor and will quickly replace your sodium-laden soy sauces. Their Thai peanut sauce is great for stir-fries and in salads. Their miso soup (I prefer mild) is a delicious cup-a-soup.

San-J International, Inc.
2880 Sprouse Drive
Richmond, VA 23231
Phone: 804-226-8333

SHELTON

Shelton poultry products are raised without antibiotics and are free-range grown. They are raised without hormones, or growth stimulants — which are common in most other commercially raised chickens and turkeys. ("All Natural" on a poultry label is defined by the Department of Agriculture as "minimally processed with no artificial ingredients." This claim on a whole bird only means that the bird has not been artificially basted, which is basically meaningless.) Shelton provides fresh poultry and other poultry-related products. Their chicken broth is excellent.

Shelton Poultry
204 Loranne
Pomona, CA 91767
Phone: 909-623-4361

SPECTRUM NATURALS

Spectrum Naturals' oils are expeller pressed without solvents. Both refined and unrefined oils are available. Their products range from oils and supplemental oils to cheese, mayonnaise, vinegars, dressings and sauces. Their brand names include Spectrum Naturals (oils), Veg-Omega, Sonnet Farms (cheese), Ayla's Organic (dressings) and Blue Banner.

Spectrum Naturals, Inc.
133 Copeland Street
Petaluma, CA 94952
Phone: 707-778-8900
Fax: 707-765-1026

SUNSPIRE

Sunspire is your answer to sugar-laden chocolate. Sunspire products contain no refined sugar and taste great. They can be purchased in carob, chocolate, mint and peanut. They provide confections and chocolate chips. They have many dairy-free products.

Sunspire
2114 Adams Avenue
San Leandro, CA 94577
Phone: 510-569-9731

VITASPELT

VitaSpelt produces some of the best whole-grain pastas. They use whole-grain spelt, which many wheat-sensitive people can tolerate. Be sure to not overcook whole-grain pasta, as that will make it mushy. They have added a new focacia bread, which can be used as an excellent pizza base. I have prepared many recipes for Vita-Spelt products.

VitaSpelt
Purity Foods Inc.
2871 West Jolly Road
Okemos, Ml 48864
Phone: 800-99-SPELT

WESTBRAE AND LITTLE BEAR

Westbrae and Little Bear are excellent brands. The company is committed to organic and low-fat products. Little Bear, under the brand Bearitos, has excellent chips, taco shells, tostada shells, popcorn, salsa, refried beans and pretzels. They also produce a licorice without refined sugar and additives. Westbrae has excellent snack food, cookies, soy milk, soy beverages and condiments.

Little Bear/Westbrae
1065 East Walnut Street
Carson, CA 90746
Phone: 310-886-8219

SUPPLEMENT MANUFACTURERS

BARLEAN'S

619-484-1035

ENZYMATIC THERAPY

800-831-7780

HERBS FOR KIDS

406-587-0111

HERBPHARM

800-348-HERB

HYLANDS (STANDARD HOMEOPATHIC COMPANY)

213-321-4284

(KYOLIC) WAKUNAGA OF AMERICA CO., LTD.

714-855-2776

RAINBOW LIGHT NUTRITIONAL SYSTEMS

800-635-1233

TRACE MINERALS

800-624-7145

Lifestyle for Health
P.O. Box 3871
Littleton, CO 80161
Phone 303-794-4477
Fax 303-794-1449

APPENDIX D
READING ^{AND} LISTENING
MATERIALS
❖❖❖

BOOKS

Anderson, Dr. Richard N.D., N.M.D., *Cleanse & Purify Thyself.* 1988.

Baker, Sidney MacDonald, M.D., *Detoxification & Health: The Key to Optimal Health.* New Canaan, CT: Keats Publishing, Inc., 1997.

Braly, James, M.D., *Dr. Braly's Food Allergy & Nutrition Revolution.* New Canaan, CT: Keats Publishing, Inc., 1992.

DeCava, Judith A., MS, LNC, *The Real Truth About Vitamins and Antioxidants.* Columbus, GA: Brentwood Academic Press, 1996.

Frähm, David & Anne, *Healthy Habits.* Colorado Springs, CO: Piñon Press, 1993.

Haas, Elson M., M.D., *The Detox Diet.* Berkeley, CA: Celestial Arts, 1996.

Hobbs, Christopher, *Natural Liver Therapy*. Capitola, CA: Botanica Press, 1988.

Jensen, Bernard, DC, *Breathe Again Naturally*. Escondido, CA: Bernard Jensen Enterprises, 1983.

Kroh, Jacqueline, M.D., *The Whole Way to Natural Detoxification*. Point Roberts, WA: Hartley & Marks Publishers, Inc., 1996.

Moore, Dr. Neecie, *The Facts About Phytochemicals*. Dallas, TX: Charis Publishing Co., 1996.

Morris, Chris, N.D., *The True Nature of Healing*. Menlo Park, CA: The Publications Group, 1997.

Murray, Michael T., N.D. and Jade Beutler, R.R.T., R.C.P., *Understanding Fats & Oils*. Encinitas, CA: Progressive Health Publishing, 1996.

Townsley, Cheryl, *Food Smart! Eat Your Way to Better Health*. Colorado Springs, CO: Piñon Press, 1994.

Townsley, Cheryl, *Kid Smart! Raising a Healthy Child*. Littleton, CO: LFH Publishing, 1996.

Townsley, Cheryl, *Revised Meals in 30 Minutes*. Littleton, CO: LFH Publishing, 1997.

TAPES

Nuggent, Dr. Steve, *Dead Doctors Don't Lie: The Rest of the Story*. Lifestyle for Health, 303-794-4477.

Townsley, Cheryl, *Cleansing made simple*. Lifestyle for Health, 303-794-4477.

Townsley, Cheryl, *Healthy Travel*. Lifestyle for Health,
303-794-4477.

Townsley, Cheryl, *It's Time to De-Stress*. Lifestyle for Health,
303-794-4477.

CATALOGS

THE COMPANY STORE

The Company Store provides quality all-cotton products.

Company Store
800-289-8508

DIAMOND ORGANIC

Diamond Organic provides organic produce by mail.

Diamond Organics
888-ORGANIC

HERITAGE STORE CATALOG

The Heritage Store provides quality, environmentally-safe products
including caster oil, ear care, essential oils, homeopathics and
much more.

Heritage Store Catalog
800-862-2923

Lifestyle for Health
P.O. Box 3871
Littleton, CO 80161
Phone 303-794-4477
Fax 303-794-1449
E-mail lfhealth@lfhealth.com
www.lfhealth.com

APPENDIX E
CHILDREN'S RESOURCES
✦✦✦

AFTER THE STORK

After the Stork offers a wide variety of children's clothing made from natural fibers.

After the Stork
1501 12th Street NW
Albuquerque, NM 87104
800-333-5437

AUTUMN HARP

Autumn Harp offers talc-free baby powder, petroleum-free jelly, petroleum-free baby oil and baby shampoo made from plant oils and herbs.

Autumn Harp
28 Rockydale Road
Bristor, VT 05443
802-453-4807

AWARENESS ENTERPRISES

Awareness Enterprises offers an audio cassette training series, *Growing a Healthy Child*, by Jennifer Beck. Containing two 90 minute tapes and a resource planner, it is designed to help parents understand the basics of health and nutrition.

Awareness Enterprises
P.O. Box 1477
Beaverton, OR 97075
503-306-0707

BABY BUNZ AND COMPANY
Baby Bunz and Company offers a wide range of natural diapering products, including Nikkys and Dovetails; 100% cotton clothing for infants, wooden baby rattles, and dolls made from all-natural materials; lambskin booties, lambskin blankets.

Baby Bunz and Company
P.O. Box 1717
Sebastopol, CA 95473
707-829-5347

BIOBOTTOMS
Biobottoms offers diapers, diaper covers, diaper duck for soiled diapers, an "It's easy to diaper with cloth" starter kit, 100% cotton clothing and shoes.

Biobottoms
Box 6009, 3820 Bodega Avenue
Petaluma, CA 94953
707-778-7945

COT'N KIDZ
Cot'n Kidz offers natural fiber clothing with standardized sizing and accessories for infants to 10 years.

Cot'n Kidz
P.O. Box 62000159
Newton, MA 01262
617-964-2686

COUNTRY COMFORT
Country Comfort offers natural baby care products.

Country Comfort
28537 Nuevo Valley Drive
P.O. Box 3
Nuevo, CA 92367
800-462-6617

EARTH'S BEST BABY FOOD
Earth's Best Baby Food offers a selection of organic baby foods
and cereals.

Earth's Best Baby Food
P.O. Box 887
Middlebury, VT 05753
800-442-4221

FAMILY CLUBHOUSE
Family Clubhouse offers natural shampoos to eliminate lice.

Family Clubhouse
6 Chiles Avenue
Asheville, NC 28803
603-675-2055

HEALTHY BABY SUPPLY COMPANY
Healthy Baby Supply Company offers a free catalog of natural
baby products or a complimentary brochure on Alternatives to Ear-
aches. Call or write Karen Kostohris at this address or number.

Healthy Baby Supply Company
323 E. Morton Street Dept. L
St. Paul, MN 55107
612-225-8535

MOTHERWEAR
Motherwear offers 100% cotton clothing and baby products.

Motherwear
P.O. Box 114
Northampton, MA 01061
413-586-3488

NATIONAL ASSOCIATION OF DIAPER SERVICES

National Association of Diaper Services helps find diaper services in specific geographical areas.

National Association of Diaper Services
2017 Walnut Street
Philadelphia, PA 19103
800-462-6237

NATURAL BABY COMPANY

Natural Baby Company offers diaper products, natural toys and other baby products.

Natural Baby Company
RDI, Box 160
Titusville, NJ 08560
800-388-BABY

NATURAL LIFESTYLE SUPPLIES

Natural Lifestyle Supplies offers natural diaper products, natural toys, baby care products and natural gift sets.

Natural Lifestyle Supplies
16 Lookout Drive
Asheville, NC 28804
800-752-2775

PERLINGER NATURALS

Perlinger Naturals offers natural baby foods.

Perlinger Naturals
238 Petaluma Avenue
Sebastopol, CA 95472
707-829-8363

SEVENTH GENERATION

Seventh Generation offers baby care products, sheets and other bedding, and natural baby wipes.

Seventh Generation
49 Hercules Drive
Colcheter, VT 05446
800-456-1177

SIMPLY PURE FOOD

Simply Pure Food offers organic strained and diced baby foods and cereals.

Simply Pure Food
RFD #3, Box 99
Bangor, ME 04401
800-426-7873

Lifestyle for Health
P.O. Box 3871
Littleton, CO 80161
Phone 303-794-4477
Fax 303-794-1449
E-mail lfhealth@lfhealth.com
www.lfhealth.com

APPENDIX F
HEALTH CARE
PROVIDERS
+++

Lifestyle for Health has compiled a national *Resource Directory* that lists health care providers, co-ops and many other products to help you on your journey toward health. For more information, or to purchase this directory, call the Lifestyle for Health office at 303-794-4477.

AMERICAN ASSOCIATION OF NATUROPATHIC PHYSICIANS

American Association of Naturopathic Physicians
2366 Eastlake Avenue, E
Seattle, WA 98102
206-323-7610

AMERICAN COLLEGE OF NURSE-MIDWIVES

American College of Nurse-Midwives
1000 Vermont Avenue, NW
Washington, DC 20005
202-728-9860

AMERICAN HOLISTIC
MEDICAL ASSOCIATION

American Holistic Medical Association
4101 Lake Boone Trail, Ste. 201
Raleigh, NC 27607
919-787-5146

AMERICAN OSTEOPATHIC ASSOCIATION

American Osteopathic Association
142 E. Ontario Street
Chicago, IL 60611
312-280-5800

BULIMIA ANOREXIA SELF-HELP, INC.

Bulimia Anorexia Self-Help, Inc.
522 N. New Ballas Road
St. Louis, MO 63141
314-567-4080

FEINGOLD ASSOCIATION OF THE U.S.

Feingold Association of the U.S.
P.O. Box 6550
Alexandria, VA 22306
703-768-3287

HOMEOPATHIC ACADEMY OF
NATUROPATHIC PHYSICIANS

Homeopathic Academy of Naturopathic Physicians
4072 9th Avenue, NE
Seattle, WA 98105
206-547-9665

INTERNATIONAL COLLEGE OF APPLIED KINESIOLOGY

International College of Applied Kinesiology
P.O. Box 905
Lawrence, KS 66044
913-0542-1801

JOHN BASTYR COLLEGE OF NATUROPATHIC MEDICINE

John Bastyr College of Naturopathic Medicine
144 NW 54th Street
Seattle, WA 98105
206-523-9585

LA LECHE LEAGUE INTERNATIONAL

La Leche League International
9816 Minneapolis Avenue
P.O. Box 1209
Franklin Park, IL 60131
800-LALECHE

Lifestyle for Health
P.O. Box 3871
Littleton, CO 80161
Phone 303-794-4477
Fax 303-794-1449
E-mail lfhealth@lfhealth.com
www.lfhealth.com

BIBLIOGRAPHY
✦✦✦

Anderson, Dr. Richard N.D., N.M.D., *Cleanse & Purify Thyself.* 1988.

Baker, Sidney MacDonald, M.D., *Detoxification & Health: The Key to Optimal Health.* New Canaan, CT: Keats Publishing, Inc., 1997.

Braly, James, M.D., *Dr. Braly's Food Allergy & Nutrition Revolution.* New Canaan, CT: Keats Publishing, Inc., 1992.

Crook, William G., M.D., *Chronic Fatigue Syndrome and the Yeast Connection.* Jackson, TN: Professional Books, 1992.

Frähm, David & Anne, *Healthy Habits.* Colorado Springs, CO: Piñon Press, 1993.

Gittleman, Ann Louise, M.S., *Beyond Pritikin.* NY, NY: Bantam Books, 1996.

Gittleman, Ann Louise, M.S., *Your Body Knows Best.* NY, NY: Pocket Books, 1997.

Golan, Ralph, M.D., *Optimal Wellness*. NY, NY: Ballantine Books, 1995.

Haas, Elson M., M.D., *The Detox Diet*. Berkeley, CA: Celestial Arts, 1996.

Hobbs, Christopher, *Natural Liver Therapy*. Capitola, CA: Botanica Press, 1988.

Jensen, Bernard, DC, *Breathe Again Naturally*. Escondido, CA: Bernard Jensen Enterprises, 1983.

Kroh, Jacqueline, M.D., *The Whole Way to Natural Detoxification*. Point Roberts, WA: Hartley & Marks Publishers, Inc., 1996.

Moore, Dr. Neecie, *The Facts About Phytochemicals*. Dallas, TX: Charis Publishing Co., 1996.

Morris, Chris, N.D., *The True Nature of Healing*. Menlo Park, CA: The Publications Group, 1997.

Murray, Michael T., N.D. and Jade Beutler, R.R.T., R.C.P., *Understanding Fats & Oils*. Encinitas, CA: Progressive Health Publishing, 1996.

Robbins, John, *May All Be Fed*. NY, NY: William Morrow & Company, Inc., 1992.

Townsley, Cheryl, *Food Smart! Eat Your Way to Better Health*. Colorado Springs, CO: Piñon Press, 1994.

Townsley, Cheryl, *Kid Smart! Raising a Healthy Child*. Littleton, CO: LFH Publishing, 1996.

Townsley, Cheryl, *Revised Meals in 30 Minutes*. Littleton, CO: LFH Publishing, 1997.

Truman, Karol K., *Feelings Buried Alive Never Die.* Las Vegas, NV: Olympus Distributing, 1995.

INDEX

✦✦✦

books, 87
breathing, 58
bronchitis, 16
bulimia, 98

C

caffeine, 34
calcium, 26
cancer, 13, 32, 41, 51
candida, 17
cardiovascular problems, 33
Cascadian Farms, 80
caster oil, 76
cellulose, 53
chewing, 34
children, 61
cholesterol, 57, 59
chronic tiredness, 35
chyme, 17
cilia, 16
cleaners, 76
coffee enema, 56, 57
colema boards, 76
Coleman, 28, 80
colitis, 32
collagen, 15
colon, 17, 55, 56
colon cleansing, 58
ConcenTrace Mineral Drops, 73
congestion, 18, 39
constipation, 32, 33, 35
cravings, 32, 35
Crohn's disease, 17

D

daily vitamins, 50

damaged fats, 33
dandelion, 56
Daniel's fast, 50
depression, 13, 32, 35
dermis, 15
despair, 25
detox baths, 46
diabetes, 13, 32
dietary changes, 45
dry hair, 33
dry nails, 33

E

eczema, 32
EFA's, 33, 50, 53, 72
elastin, 15
electro magnetic fields, 30
EMF's, 30
emotional toxins, 19
emphysema, 15
enema bags, 76
enemas, 56
energy, 20
environmental toxins, 20
Enzymatic Therapy, 85
enzymes, 17, 20, 31, 50, 53, 71, 72
epidermis, 15
Epson salts, 47
esophagus, 16
essential fatty acids, 15
exercise, 59, 65

F

fasting, 49
fatigue, 32, 33

fear, 19
Feingold Association, 98
fennel, 56
fiber, 31, 50, 51, 71
fibromyalgia, 13, 51, 19
fluorescent lights, 30
food cravings, 32
formaldehyde, 30
Frontier Herbs, 80
fungus, 17

G
gallbladder, 16
gallbladder flush, 57
gastrointestinal tract, 16
GI tract, 16, 51
ginger root baths, 47
glyco sugars, 52
glyconutrients, 71
glyconutrition, 50, 52, 72
glycoproteins, 52, 53
good health, 14
green produce, 26
greens powders, 49
grief, 25
guilt, 25

H
hatred, 25
healing crisis, 41
heart disease, 13, 32
herbal tea baths, 48
Herbs for Kids, 85
Heritage Store, 76
high blood pressure, 33
Homeopathic Academy, 98

homeopathics, 64
homeostasis, 18
Horizon, 81
hormones, 20
hostility, 25
hotels, 30
hydrochloric acid, 17
Hylands, 85
hypo-adrenia, 35

I
immune weakness, 33
implants, 41
inadequate finances, 25
indigestion, 33
inflexibility, 25
insecurity, 25
insomnia, 32
ionic minerals, 54
iron, 26
irritable bowel syndrome, 17
irritation, 25

K
kidneys, 18
Kinesiology, 99
KyoGreen, 49, 73
Kyolic, 85

L
La Leche League, 99
lactase, 53
lactobacilli, 51
large intestine, 16
larynx, 15
laundry products, 76

Y
yeast, 17

Z
zeolite, 75

BOOKS

LIFESTYLE FOR HEALTH COOKBOOK
by Cheryl Townsley
Delicious health food including: 8 weeks of menus and grocery lists, over 180 recipes with nutritional analysis, alternatives for sugar, white flour, fat, salt and dairy, many references and much more.
Wire spiral bound $24.00

REVISED MEALS IN 30 MINUTES
by Cheryl Townsley
Learn the best foods your body needs for weight, mood and energy balance. Tasty recipes help you cook once and eat many times. Recommended supplements for busy people and a section on making cooking fun make this book a winner. $15.00

COOKBOOK SPECIAL —
Set of both cookbooks $35.00

KID SMART!
by Cheryl Townsley
Information, strategies and recipes to help transition any person — child or adult — from the average American diet to a healthier diet. Includes information on natural alternatives to antibiotics and solutions for common ailments. $15.00

FOOD SMART!
by Cheryl Townsley
Cheryl shares her story from suicide attempt and near death to health. Learn how to become emotionally and mentally, as well as physically, healthy. A great story that provides practical insight, along with practical helps to health. $14.00

GET SMART SPECIAL
Get both *Kid Smart!* and *Food Smart!* for one great price! $25.00

RETURN TO PARADISE
by Cheryl Townsley
Is your life scattered with tiredness and sickness? Are you living a life of lack and dissatisfaction? *Return to Paradise* brings insight on these modern death grips. God created a beautiful garden for mankind. Adam and Eve had perfect health, perfect provision and God–given purpose ... You can too! $12.00

HEALTHY HABITS
by Dave and Anne Frähm
Easy ways to get started on your path to better health and the documented reasons for each of these healthy habits. $14.00

UNDERSTANDING FATS & OILS
by Michael Murray, N.D., and Jade Beutler, R.R.T., R.C.P.
This is the best book I have read to help you understand the differences between good and bad fats. Has recipes for flaxseed oil. $5.00

YOUR BODY KNOWS BEST
by Ann Louise Gittleman
The best book to help you understand metabolic profiling from a balanced expert in the nutritional field. $6.50

NEWSLETTER

LIFESTYLE FOR HEALTH
12 pages of nutritional information, recipes, health updates, new product reviews and a touch of humor.
6 issues/year $16.00

SOFTWARE

DINNER!
AND LIFESTYLE FOR HEALTH COOKBOOK
This computer software is easy to use and a real time saver! Includes 16 weeks of menus, recipes, grocery lists and nutritional charts — *plus* the capability to add and analyze your own recipes.

Available for IBM & Macintosh computers. System requirements — 386 or higher IBM compatible PC • 4MB RAM • Microsoft Windows 3.1 or higher • requires 7.5 MB hard drive space

Add $4.00 shipping/handling per item to order instead of 15%.

Please specify MAC or IBM PC on order form. $65.00

SUPPLEMENTS

MANNACLEANSE
Our favorite daily cleanse in caplet form. $38.00

CONCENTRACE MINERAL DROPS
The best value and source for mineral supplementation. $10.50

BARLEAN'S FLAX OIL
12 oz. $12.00

DIGEST–A–MEAL ENZYMES
$26.00

TOTAL FLORA SUPPORT
Friendly probiotic support. $26.00

PHYT–ALOE
Plant phytochemicals and antioxidant support for a strong immune system. $38.00

PHYTO–BEARS
Phyt–Aloe in a gummy–bear form, a real favorite with kids of all ages!
$19.50

PLUS
Endocrine, adrenal and hormone system support. $38.00

SPORT
Supports lean tissue development and muscle recovery after sports workouts. $35.00

MAN–ALOE
Supports cellular communication.
$38.00

METABOLIC PROFILE #1
Multi–Vitamin $44.00

METABOLIC PROFILE #2
Multi–Vitamin $44.00

METABOLIC PROFILE #3
Multi–Vitamin $44.00

KYO–GREEN
Our favorite greens food drink.
$28.00

All prices subject to change.

IT'S FREE!

To Obtain Your FREE Copy of Cheryl Townsley's Lifestyle for Health Newsletter

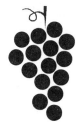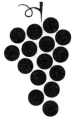

CALL 303-794-4477

AUTHOR
✦✦✦

Cheryl Townsley is the founder of Lifestyle for Health, a company dedicated to helping people restore their total health to its full God-given potential. Cheryl has been a keynote speaker for national seminars, conferences and trade associations. She has been featured on hundreds of national and international television and radio programs.

Cheryl is known for her insight and humor, evident as she provides practical strategies to restore health. All, from individuals to whole families, will find opportunity to step into health with hope and encouragement with Cheryl.

Since 1991, Cheryl has published an international, bimonthly newsletter: the *Lifestyle for Health Newsletter.* In addition she has published five books: *Food Smart!, Lifestyle for Health* cookbook, *Meals in 30 Minutes, Kid Smart!* and *Return to Paradise.*

Cheryl resides in Denver, Colorado, with her husband, Forest, and their daughter, Anna.